# INCISIONS

An insider's guide to finding the best surgeon for your condition.

**Read this before you go under the knife!**

Dr. SAURABH MISRA

STARDOM BOOKS

www.StardomBooks.com

**STARDOM BOOKS**
A Division of Stardom Publishing
and infoYOGIS Technologies.
105-501 Silverside Road
Wilmington, DE 19809

FIRST EDITION OCTOBER 2022

STARDOM BOOKS

A Division of Stardom Alliance
105-501 Silverside Road Wilmington, DE 19809,
USA

www.stardombooks.com

Stardom Books, United States
Stardom Books, India

The author and publishers have made all reasonable efforts to contact copyright-holders for permission, and apologize for any omissions or errors in the form of credits given. Corrections may be made to future editions.

Dr. Saurabh Misra

p. 224
cm. 13.5 X 21.5

Category:
MED085000 - Medical : Surgery – General
MED000000 - Medical : General

ISBN:  978-1-957456-14-0

# DEDICATION

My Father, Late Shri Kirti Prakash Misra

# CONTENTS

# ACKNOWLEDGMENTS

My sincere thanks to my wife, Seema, who bore the brunt of this book by just being by my side all the time and providing me with the support and relaxation that only an anaesthetist could provide to a surgeon, on a very bad day at work. To my mother, Dr Madhuri Misra, who is always a literary inspiration behind all my idiotic ideas and writings.

To my kids, Shreyas and Arundhati, for being the kids that everyone would want to have!

Sincere gratitude to all my friends and colleagues who put their hearts and souls into providing the input into relevant chapters, so that the right information goes to the patients. They could have used their precious time to do something else.

Sincere thanks to my publishers and editors for pushing me on and understanding my time constraints, especially Raam Anand, who had faith in me and thought I could produce something like a book!

And finally, the writer and poet in me who needed an avenue for expression!

Furthermore, my sincere thanks to:

Orthopaedic Surgery - Dr Pradeep Kocheeppan, D.Ortho, DNB (Orthopaedic surgery), Fellowship in Knee and shoulder surgeries, Senior Consultant Orthopaedic surgeon, Apollo Hospitals, Bangalore.

Neurosurgery: Dr Vikram Kamath, MD, DM. Neurology, Senior Consultant Neurologist, Apollo Hospitals, Bangalore.

: Dr Arun L Naik, MS, MCh. Neurosurgery, Senior Consultant, Neurosurgeon, Apollo Hospitals, Bangalore.

Cardio thoracic surgery: Dr Satyaki Nambala, MS, MCh, Cardiothoracic surgery, Senior Consultant, Cardiothoracic surgeon, Apollo Hospitals, Bangalore.

Surgical Oncology: Dr Anil Kamath, MS, MCh. (Surgical Oncology), DNB (Surgical Oncology), Senior Consultant, Surgical Oncology and Robotic oncology, Apollo Hospitals, Bangalore.

Gynae and Obs surgery: Dr Rani Bhat, MS. OBG, MRCOG, Fellowship in Gyne-Oncology, Senior Consultant, Gynaeoncology, Apollo Hospitals, Bangalore.

Urology: Dr Sreedhar Reddy, MS, MCh, Urology, Senior Consultant Urologist, Apollo Hospitals, Bangalore.

Otolaryngology: Dr Satish Nair, MS. ENT, Senior Consultant ENT and head and neck surgeon, Apollo Hospitals, Bangalore.

Ophthalmologist: Dr Shalini Shetty, MS, FRCS, Ophthalmologist, Senior Consultant Ophthalmologist, Apollo Hospitals, Bangalore.

Plastic surgery: Dr Naveen Rao, MS, MCh, Plastic surgery, Senior Consultant Plastic surgeon, Apollo Hospitals, Bangalore.

# INTRODUCTION

In January 2019, my father developed chest pain, and I took him to the ER in the hospital where I worked. He was evaluated, and the ER physician broke the news to me that he was having a Myocardial Infarction (heart attack). His blood pressure and pulse rate were fine, which meant that I could take a few moments to reflect on which cardiology colleague to talk to for further management. We had roughly 15 cardiologists and five units to choose from. This was a difficult decision, perhaps more difficult than getting him to the ER and getting the correct diagnosis! I had a wonderful working relationship with my cardiology colleagues, having worked in the hospital for more than 14 years. It was an extremely difficult decision to make.

After much thought, I zeroed in on a couple of colleagues who had consistently shown good results. I had not heard many buzzes about their practice either. Most controversial events in the Operating Room (OR) or other places like the Intensive Care Units (ICUs) would be discussed in the 'Mortality meets' or the 'Board rooms,' so I would have known.

On the one hand, I had a slightly younger colleague in my group, who was close to me, and we would regularly meet at clubs for drinks.

On the other hand, there was an older gentleman who was a retired professor with thousands of angioplasties and years of experience under his belt. It became slightly easier to decide because I knew their results were comparable.

My decision was based on approachability. I chose my friend over the more experienced colleague. Thankfully, my father's procedure went fine, with the stenting of two coronary vessels. I have never regretted my decision.

However, when I sat outside the Cathlab during the procedure, I wondered would go through a patient's mind when they did not have the same knowledge which I had. How would they choose their surgeon or caregiver?

How would they decide on the surgeon without knowing the disease, the procedure, the hospital, the surgeon's outcomes, and the surgeon's skill level (in my case, a physician)? It is even more difficult at the time of emergencies when there is little or no time to think and consult your family or the GP.

Many years ago, at the beginning of my career as a bariatric surgeon, I received a call in my clinic. It was a pleasant young man who asked for an appointment for his mother, who weighed 145 kgs. They wanted to get a bariatric procedure done. He was a doctor from a neighbouring state.

I gladly accepted and wished to have a physical consultation. However, on seeing her, my heart sank. She was just 1.4 metres tall, had diabetes, and even had trouble walking 10 metres. All the red flags in my mind went up! She was a bad case, and I did not have enough skills to tackle her case. I asked him what made him approach me. He answered that his friend had seen me speaking at a conference a few months ago and had referred me. I then referred him to a high-volume centre out of state, and she did well subsequently.

Today, things are different; we have enough experience and well-oiled machinery in place to tackle such cases. But I wonder sometimes, how could a doctor not know that I was just not up to it.

I deduced that it was the combination of factors, including the referral from a friend, our good rapport during the first conversation, and a fairly untarnished image on the internet, which may have made him seek my help. But then, is that enough to make him trust his mother's life in my hands? Is there a better way to understand and make informed decisions in this regard?

For the average uninformed and unconnected patient, such a scenario would present a double whammy. On the one hand, the patient has to face the ensuing emotional turmoil when the attending physician tells them about the diagnosis and need for a procedure. On the other hand, the attendant of the patient would be faced with the dilemma of first verifying the diagnosis and the decision. Then, the question would arise as to who is the right person to tackle the issue.

The problem does not end here! The first human reaction in such a case would be denial. So typically, when confronted with a diagnosis that would need surgery or a procedure, the first reaction would be the denial of the diagnosis and the whole process itself. This denial could last for an hour or as long as a day or a week. I have seen multiple cases of this reaction play out, resulting in the patient's health going downhill. I recall an incident where a young person with abdominal pain was diagnosed to have abdominal tuberculosis. His situation worsened over months due to inaction, and his family finally had to return to the hospital with him in a hopeless and dying state. This reaction is not unique and has left me wondering if the information system we have today is adequate.

When we investigated the case further, we found out that the relatives were worried about the exposure to the coronavirus in the hospital. They did not want him to be further afflicted and thus did not get him admitted to the hospital. The corona epidemic has made things worse. For the first time, the doctors are at a loss for words about the epidemic itself and what to do about it! However, the mortality rate due to corona is about 1.7 percent and pales in comparison to the deaths due to non-corona cases because of nonavailability/denial of treatment.

In the aforementioned case, the patient's family did not know that the hospital had invested hugely in the infrastructure changes to keep the non-corona patients safe from exposure to the disease. They did not know that the fever clinic and the corona wards were segregated from the non-corona cases.

At the bottom of this issue is a "lack of information and clarity" about what happens once you are admitted. Who will treat you? How will the patient be managed? How much will it cost? And finally, how long will the patient be in the hospital? The answers to all these questions are never straightforward, and more so in case of emergencies.

The junior-most member in the unit is usually on call at night, and he still would not have acquired the necessary diplomacy and polish to deal with different sorts of patients and their relatives. He is badly overworked and frustrated with the continuous calls and would not have managed to eat anything on most call days. He will be rude because he is exhausted and does not have the patience to answer the seemingly foolish questions of the relatives. I do not justify or endorse such behaviour by any means. Such incidents are always taken seriously, and the doctors have always been given an earful by me. But most patients don't let it out and quietly walk out of the hospital at the end of the treatment. My aim in writing this book is to put down their point of view, let patients understand the situations in which they work, and empathetically relate to them. In other words, I want to convey what goes into making a good surgeon!

What makes one a surgeon? When you meet a surgeon, you will realize that they are doctors who seem to belong to a slightly different species compared to the other usual doctors. They are somewhat more polished (not all), a little better dressed (usually, but not all of them), and are always arrogant. I have undergone years of training and worked with many surgeons. I have come to like a few of them and dislike the most of them! This made me look at myself and wonder, what have I become?

I really can't relate to any one surgeon, but I can see many of my teachers in me, and it is embarrassing to note that I might, at times, become the teacher I most disliked.

The effect and the stress of surgical training are too much to bear, and you come out of the training period a different person from the one who entered the training period. I remember my first few days in the surgical ward. It was nothing like Grey's Anatomy (the TV show), which I had seen earlier. The smell of decaying diabetic ulcers and urine would be overwhelming, and it stayed with you for days and haunted you when you came back to your quarters and tried to eat your food.

Your clothes would smell like a dead fish that had been rotting for a long time. Then there were the call days where you would be the lowest ranking "officer" in the whole platoon of people. There would be hours and hours of ER duty, where you would stitch wounds and resurrect the dead and dying! The worst part of surgical emergencies were never the buried appendicitis or the faeces pouring out of the intestines. It was always the young people who came in with burn injuries or head injuries caused by accidents. These patients posed a different challenge to a young, unprepared soul who was a poet at heart and got a prize for creative writing! The burns were either self-inflicted or revenge-induced, and usually, the patients were young girls. Some of them were just married! The sounds of their painful screams and the sight of their peeling skin accompanied by the stench of burning skin can be so overwhelming that you would want to leave or puke. You would want to go away and never come back!

The head injuries would present violent movements with bleeding, vomiting, and disorientation. Usually, if you examined them for more than five minutes, you would risk being vomited upon, and then the smell will linger on you for hours. The dreamer within me stopped dreaming and stayed put as this was a reality far deeper than anything I was prepared for. I would always ask myself, where was the surgeon this training promised to make me?

Then there would be the excitement of surgery when the real stuff would begin, and we got an idea of what would be our actual profession—The surgical stuff! Mostly in the early part of the training, it usually meant opening up the abdomen and closing it.

We had to ensure that the counts for the gauze and the abdominal packs would tally and that the drains were placed properly in the abdomen. It was never easy in those days, and it is never easy today. With the number of surgical packs lost in the abdomen reaching 1 in 5500 to 7000 surgeries every year worldwide, and increasing litigations, the work of the first-year resident has reached higher levels. I know a few consultants who have been attending court meetings for the last ten years without any resolution for the same cause!

The life of a resident is akin to a battered and bruised soldier.

Usually, the first-year resident returns to his den way past midnight with no food and sleeps for a few hours only to be woken again a couple of times more in the night. They usually get only two to three hours of sleep for many days at a stretch. The only incentive would be a surgery or two to be done independently at night. These surgeries would help keep his self-respect at an acceptable level.

The days are never easy when you are on 'rounds' with a senior Professors who is also probably dissatisfied with his 'government' job. He is further frustrated as he cannot fulfil the ever-increasing demands of a family that doesn't listen to him anymore. He is often irritated and impatient and lives in the bubble of institutional life; more often then not, he only gets a resident to command and abuse. From his point of view, he is simply bored of this mundane life. The same type of patients come each year, with the same surgeries happening yearly. He wants to see one resident who would shine almost immediately as soon as he comes into the ward. If he finds one such resident, he can then leave the aftercare of the patients to that resident and rely on him for the next three years. Most of the senior doctors with the exception of a few (I had the pleasure of being with at least one such professor who was a teacher more then a surgeon, Dr KC Vyas.) does not have the patience to spend time with the new residents, understand them, and help them become the best they can be. Instead, most bosses are quick to judge and make assumptions based on how they were as residents and fail to fulfil their commitment as teachers and guides. It is often a waste of talent and resources when many wonderful minds pass the final surgical exams with little confidence and self-respect.

But I am told that things have changed and better days are ahead. Today, as a teacher, I try to understand the new resident and make the best use of his talents. At the very least, I try not to humiliate them. There is not much that can be given as 'hands-on' to these young people in a corporate hospital, but I try to tell them how to be safe surgeons and have the right attitude. But more often than not, the same story is repeated. As super-specialist minimal access surgery teachers, we train students who are already surgeons and have their degrees and licenses to practice surgery. But their training as PG students would open up like a book to me. Most students are scarred for life, and their attitudes are written in stone by their earlier teachers. Some of the students learn and understand. But the best students are the ones who quickly adapt and unlearn what they had learned earlier. By encouraging them to ask questions, I get to know their keenness to learn. I have found that their malleability is the key to becoming excellent surgeons.

As these young surgeons grow from residents to senior residents/registrars and later as fellows and associates, they learn a lot and change into completely different individuals from the ones they were when they passed their PG exams. These are the surgeons who would finally interact with the general public as consultants in hospitals. This metamorphosis has always fascinated me in more ways than one. At times, I get scared to see their confidence only to realise that I am seeing myself in them!

This book is all about the patients and their surgeons. I have realised that all the while when I was training, and later, I only looked at myself and forgot about the patient and their near and dear ones. I have often heard surgeons complain about their practice never taking off despite the good training and credentials.

It made me wonder what made one surgeon click and not the others. Then after months of research and multiple questions in Quora and Survey Monkey, I concluded that the one thing that distinguished a successful surgeon from others was the 'connect.' It was about empathy. That connection was critical! From the patient's point of view, that was enough.

But is that the only way to get the right surgeon? After all, patients are paying for the services rendered, and they expect the right person for the right job!

Keeping that in mind, I embarked on the journey to create a model where you are likely to get the correct answers if applied to in the real-life situations. Good surgical outcomes are not only about smooth-talking clinicians but beyond that and much more.

In the chapters that follow, we will explore how surgeons are created in the different specialities and super-specialist fields. We will also try to guide you in the correct decision-making procedures for the best clinical outcomes for you and your near and dear ones when it comes to choosing the right surgeon for the right job.

# 1
# A GOOD DOCTOR

As I watch the HBO drama, 'The Knick,' suggested by my good friend Anil, the flamboyant and arrogant surgeon makes a statement on the screen "You are legitimising surgery, moving it out of the barbershops and into the future." Thackery tells this to his predecessor in the first episode, reminiscing on his start at the hospital. "I want to be a part of it." The genera of surgeons across the world were born about that time. Our forefathers (the barbers) had no pride!

Modern surgery was born the day it moved from the marketplace to the operation theatre. Along with this move came the seduction and the arrogance of being a surgeon. The field of 'surgery' has been refined throughout the next century by the 'real guys' of the medical profession (sorry, the other 'people'). The whole show gives us surgeons the goosebumps. Nothing about the arrogance and the panache has changed since then.

Show me a surgeon who does not display anger and a childish demeanour: he is either an unsuccessful surgeon or at least not the guy who makes enough money! If you look at a typical medical board meeting attended by a mix of surgeons and physicians, the surgeons are the ones who are more inappropriate and brash, and they are usually the first ones to walk out following a disagreement in contrast to the physicians, who are cuter and more articulate. Even at renowned hospitals, the money squeezing and bribes shown on The Knick may have happened. Medical Chaos and Crime, a 1910 book authored by a physician who had worked at New York and Washington Heights hospitals, made a stir by claiming to detail extreme hospital misconduct—drunk night nurses, unscrupulous superintendents, and incompetently trained surgeons.

Few things may have changed since then! Except, in a more polished way, we continue to deliver mixed satisfaction rates to patients. You may not encounter drunk nurses these days but the corporatization of the health system has led to a new and more cautious approach toward the hospitals and patients have become more suspicious toward the treatments and outcomes.

A typical example of this is what happened in an Agra hospital in June 2021: the doctors were blamed by the relatives of the 22 patients who died allegedly due to lack of oxygen, which was said to have been turned off as part of a 'mock drill.' This was at the height of the COVID pandemic and it was not the fault of the treating doctors. The decision regarding the disruption of the oxygen supply for five minutes was taken by the owner of the hospital. The burden of surgical intervention on public health systems will continue to expand with the rising prevalence of severe accidents, malignancies, and cardiovascular diseases.

Surgical intervention is sometimes the sole way to relieve impairments and lower the risk of mortality from common diseases. Surgical interventions account for an estimated 13% of the world's total disability-adjusted life years, with millions of individuals undergoing treatment each year. While surgical operations are meant to save lives, poor surgical care can result in serious consequences, given the prevalence of surgery.

It is important to understand the progress of surgery in modern times, especially as the American College of Surgeons prepares to hold its 100th annual conference in San Francisco. Surgeons were represented as having masculine type A personalities some decades ago, which remains unchanged, and a few surgeons have been termed as spoiled brats of the hospital. Surgeons were regarded and respected, and their autonomy and power were assumed. Patients almost never questioned the treatment plan. With strong dyadic mentor-mentee interactions, the training model was pyramidal. The approach to surgical education was "see one, do one, teach one." Being there to personally manage situations in the hospital and being 'on call' every other night provided the requisite experience. The majority of operations were open surgical procedures performed in the main operating room, with surgeons frequently manning multiple rooms. Surgical patients usually had to stay in the hospital for a long time before fully recovering. Inpatient services were often substantial, with 50 to 60 patients under each service. The practice of surgery has changed dramatically during the last several decades. With the entry of more women and minorities into the surgical specialty, the field is becoming more diversified.

The surgical techniques have been transformed from 'open' to laparoscopic or keyhole surgery to robotic-assisted surgeries. The next decade may see an autonomous robot doing basic surgeries with precision and uniform results, while human intervention may only be required in a handful of the more complex cases.

As I write this, millions of dollars are spent on machine learning and AI, which have the potential to transform the landscape of surgery. Despite the fact that some surgeons believe they are not as respected by the general community as they once were, many have improved their work-life balance.

Patients are more inquisitive about the results, duration of hospital stay, and surgeon's volume of cases. Surgeons have less authority and are held responsible for higher standards in terms of revenue cycles, policies, and regulations. The corporate culture has brought about a lot of positive changes in the healthcare system. These changes are not necessarily surgeon-friendly, but they are definitely patient- and hospital-centric. Operations include open and minimally invasive surgeries, which take place in both the operating rooms and in the outpatient departments.

Hospital inpatient services are smaller with a significant turnover rate, and the length of stay following surgical procedures is shorter.

A higher emphasis is placed on patient safety and results. In addition to surgeons and surgical trainees, multidisciplinary care teams increasingly include a variety of healthcare practitioners. The move from individual surgeon-based care to team-based care has been a significant transformation in surgical care delivery. Expanding the care teams to include nurses, nurse practitioners, physician assistants, pharmacists, and other healthcare practitioners, in addition to the surgeons, has improved patient safety and results. The focus has shifted away from the surgeon's requirements and toward the needs of the patient. Patient satisfaction and results are improved by scheduling visits and therapies around people and their conditions.

Furthermore, focusing solely on physician-centred outcomes is no longer the optimal way to provide patient care. Patients require more than just good surgical outcomes. They require TLC now! Oddly, healthcare services have now become the Healthcare Industry and can easily be confused with the Hospitality Industry. Just when the healthcare industry was struggling with the nomenclature, it was put in the gambit of the consumer law. This broke the fine fabric of patient-clinician relationships and patients were treated like consumers. Reprimanding the surgeons for a few wrong outcomes was never going to be a good idea. The clinicians became afraid and the patients became impatient. Thus started the culture of defensive medicine where the patient was burdened with a lot of unnecessary tests and subjected to surgery in borderline indications.

Patients too responded in the most aggressive and sometimes in the most passive-aggressive ways. One of our patients did not turn up for surgery because his car got dented in the hospital car park! While another patient was hysterical at the end of the successful surgery because his pillow cover had a hole and was not changed until the next morning.

A lot of my surgical colleagues are struggling with lawsuits due to billing-related issues that have nothing to do with the final outcome of the surgery.

Readmission rates have decreased as a result of the team approach, which includes thorough planning before surgery along with discharge planning, seeing patients immediately after release, and even phoning patients at home. Teamwork is vital because it allows the surgeon to focus on the indication for intervention, the treatment or operation, and the prevention and treatment of complications. Most patients are happy with the team treatment. Over the last few decades, the practice of contemporary surgery has changed dramatically.

What criteria does one use to determine what is wrong with a patient? To put it another way, how do you make a diagnosis? Doctors and surgeons have attempted to address that question throughout the history of medicine. They have always been confronted with the patient's dread since the outset. Anyone who believes their time is coming to an end wants to hear how it will happen from their doctor.

Is there any hope left? How much longer do I have? Will I be in pain? To intelligently respond to these inquiries, one must first understand the patient's situation. Doctors were better at it than anybody else since they had seen more diseases and problems throughout their lifetimes. Surgeons and detectives both appear to approach their cases in the same way: they both look for contradictions, generate theories, reason rationally, and deliberate. Signs and symptoms (or clues) are elicited (deduced) and decoded. The value of a great surgeon's effectiveness cannot be overstated. The word "brilliant" literally means "very bright, wonderful," and it is used to describe someone who is extremely intelligent and skilful. Evidence reveals that a few distinct characteristics are associated with brilliance and success in life. All highly successful people, regardless of their career, have a set of characteristics. It has been discovered that there are a few common personality traits that relate to world-class performances.

These traits pertain to the cognitive, psychomotor, and affective domains and guide human success in almost all fields. Evidence also identifies "smart" people. "Surgeon" is a term used to describe people with exceptional surgical skills or operative abilities.

They are daring and dexterous enough to deal with difficult situations or instances that are incredibly challenging. They have great preoperative workup and diagnostic abilities because they know when to operate and when not to operate. Their operational results are unrivalled, and their postoperative care is flawless, resulting in few or no postoperative complications. They are also regarded as the most skilled and brilliant surgeons among their peers. There have been studies that show a positive correlation between spatial ability and psychomotor skill or aptitude and improved surgical performance in clinical situations; however, aside from anecdotes, very few studies have focused on the personality traits of surgeons, which may be important for becoming a successful and brilliant surgeon. There is evidence that a unique surgical personality exists. The underlying technical aspects of the personality do play a key influence in being brilliant, according to studies that have discovered the personality traits or attributes of clever surgeons. The study's goal was to investigate the idea of a "bright surgeon" by determining the most prevalent personality features of these surgeons who were considered the finest among their peers.

Mental domain, psychological and emotional domain, social domain, mechanical domain, and structural strength domain were the five basic topics that predominantly defined the brilliance of surgeons.

Domain of the Mind refers to the ongoing learning successes of surgical education (cognitive domain). It is made up of a number of key components that are listed in order of preference. These are the strong pillars that sustain a surgeon's multidimensional framework of brilliance.

Each domain was further broken into several sub-themes, which also showed the number of times each participant cited the same characteristic.

When addressing surgical crises, problem-solving ability, particularly thinking on one's feet, is an important aspect of decision-making. When it comes to making a judgment on a multidimensional clinical issue, excellent surgeons are always thorough and detail-oriented.

Reflection with understanding and analysis of what has been done in order to effectively learn from the experiences leads to constant self-improvement, which is a vital characteristic of exceptional surgeons who are never happy with routine work. Their drive to study the most up-to-date information necessitates the habit of following a continual learning process in surgical education. The majority of them were self-aware of their limits, which they considered crucial to their desire to develop. The majority of them were careful and well-organised, and they were ready to take on challenging situations. I always felt brilliant surgeons are born! The others are also there to complete the whole picture and then there are the ones who will make a living and not a career.

All of them are an important part of complete surgical coverage. As I look at my developmental stages, I became increasingly comfortable with my Minimal Access surgical skills and later on became confident in two key areas—Minimal-access Bariatric Surgery and Upper GI surgery and minimal-access complex hernia surgeries. Much of my general surgery practice did not give me the high anymore, and rightly so, as a lot of my surgical colleagues make a living out of the mundane stuff! Not everyone needs to become a Rafael Nadal or a Novak Djokovic of the surgical field.

The other attributes of a good surgeon include being goal-oriented, forecasting the optimal treatment outcome, participating in research, and being flexible. Although these are the less commonly mentioned attributes, they are nevertheless crucial in reaching brilliance in the art of surgery. Brilliant surgeons possess strong leadership characteristics and like leading their teams. It is important that they be leaders in their field and their environment.

They also must have excellent communication skills, which is another important skill for surgeons.

They must be able to take the initiative. They are dependable and straightforward; they are trustworthy in their actions and provide team members with unrestricted guidance. Because of the need to operate with incredibly sharp tools, a great surgeon must have immaculate hand dexterity in synchronisation with economy of motions.

Without perfection and accuracy, the outcomes might be catastrophic. Dexterity was the most often mentioned domain among our responders in the survey that we conducted. Enhanced psychomotor abilities in the form of outstanding surgical and tissue handling skills were rated by all of the doctors as a crucial aptitude for success in operational surgery.

Highly successful surgeons are unique because of their mechanical labor propensity and exceptional hand dexterity. To sustain the lengthy, irregular working hours and attend to the odd-time crises, a surgeon needs enormous physical vitality, stamina, and physical effort. According to the responders, excellent surgeons have a plethora of these skills and requirements.

I know a lot of surgeons who were simply let down by the intention-tremors (involuntary shaking) of their hands. When they were young, they somehow managed to get by, but later in life, it became impossible to operate. They just left the surgical practice to go into teaching and administration.

The ability to face obstacles head-on was the most prevalent characteristic among exceptional surgeons. To withstand these demands, he/she needs a high sense of self-worth. Dedication, persistence, patience, mental endurance, and objectivity were the next most often occurring attributes that were thought to have substantially contributed to their lifetime success as outstanding surgeons. Empathy, selflessness, and humility were also discovered to be significant humanistic characteristics in their personalities. The majority felt that being courageous and having effective emergency response skills are characteristics of their identity.

Enthusiasm, confidence, calmness, self-reliance, dynamism, and competitive spirit were seen as necessary characteristics for exceptional surgeons.

The terms "good surgeon," "excellent surgery," and "good surgical abilities" have long piqued the curiosity of critics. It has always been a difficult question to answer. However, these three elements cannot be discussed in isolation. If the outcome of a surgery is poor, one cannot call the surgical skill good, even if it is exceptional when seen in isolation.

To reach brilliance, one must evaluate the issue holistically and recognise the numerous components of a great surgeon operating in a surgical environment. The surgeon has a cult image of brilliance as a result of his/her ability to accomplish highly specialised jobs with exceptional physical dexterity. In actuality, a great surgeon requires not just exceptional physical agility, but also a variety of other cognitive and non-cognitive characteristics that are equally important in his quest for perfection, not to mention his physical ability to undergo physical abuse due to long hours of surgery. Patients began to receive increasingly sophisticated elective surgical therapies as antisepsis and anaesthesia became more refined and widely available. Surgery is no longer limited to amputations and abscess draining. Tonsillectomies, hernia repairs, and appendectomies were the most frequent surgeries performed at the Pennsylvania Hospital by 1925.

Modern surgery gave doctors the ability to operate on people voluntarily and return them to their premorbid state safely and painlessly. As a result, surgeons were no longer just last-resort physicians to whom patients turned for life-saving but frequently morbid surgeries. Furthermore, surgical therapy is now being practiced by an expanding number of young, aggressive, particularly qualified physicians who provided surgical care to patients for a growing range of illnesses. The rise in the number and the variety or scope of optional, revenue-generating operations necessitated the development of a professional code of ethics.

In 1913, members of the American College of Surgeons signed a commitment pledging to "put the welfare and rights of my patient above everything else." It is valid till today! This code aided surgeons in their actions and increased public trust by ensuring patients that the purpose of surgical therapy was improved health, not increased professional revenue.

While advances in aesthetic methods and minimally invasive procedures have allowed many more surgeries to be conducted with shorter hospital stays or even as outpatient treatments, the overall cost of surgical care is rising. As a result, the specialty of surgery has been the target of employer and government efforts to contain rising medical expenses by extending utilisation review and managed care programs to a higher extent than the other medical specialties have been.

Managed care insurers frequently shift the financial risk of healthcare usage to physicians and institutions, among other cost-control techniques, in order to incentivise cost-effective treatment. Many patients and clinicians are worried that because of the relationship between finance and service supply, necessary and effective services may be withheld, causing a conflict between a physician's financial interest and a patient's health interest.

It is a double whammy for the surgeons: while the patients demand top-notch results, the insurers and the hospitals want to cut costs and pay less and less to the clinician. This tension has the potential to erode the patients' faith in their doctors' judgments, posing a major danger to the doctor-patient relationship.

As a result, despite the ability of surgeons and other physicians to extend and/or improve life to a greater extent than they had in the past, the connection between surgeons and their patients is as tense as it has ever been.

Despite the fact that the majority of patients continue to have trust in their surgeons, public opinion has generally turned against doctors and surgeons in general. It is the players behind the curtain who are responsible for all the elements of the modern hospital, such as the billing, infrastructure, food, and operations.

These people are invisible. The only visible people are the patients and the doctors. So, whenever there is an event in the hospital that is unrelated to the surgery, the only person who takes the blame is the doctor, right from the poor air conditioning to the dripping toilet tap.

### How to choose your surgeon?

In spite of the above-mentioned criteria that are accepted worldwide, the question of choosing the right surgeon remains. Is there any definite way of knowing 'Who is the right surgeon for me?' A very difficult question indeed! It is really difficult for an average patient to answer this question. While most of them would go to the humble family physician next door, the more tech savvy patients resort to Uncle Google.

Sometimes, despite all the due diligence, patients develop complications and bear huge healthcare costs. The surgeon-patient relationship has been put under unprecedented stress due to changes in the healthcare system's structure. Knot-tying and sewing skills are useful, and some of today's most smart and famous surgeons were not recognised for their dexterity as medical students or junior surgical residents. The key characteristics, which surpass the little disparities in dexterity among most medical students, are: Intelligence, Professionalism, Conscientiousness, Inventiveness, Courage, and Tenacity on behalf of your patients. It takes a lifetime to become a good surgeon.

As a surgical mentor, I see a lot of young surgeons who come and get trained with us; a few of them require to be trained vigorously, a few require to be reminded of the skills taught in the laboratory, and yet a few of them would have made excellent veterinary surgeons who could remove a large volume of scybalous polythene from a cow's rectum or stomach rather than general surgeons who operated on human beings.

The most crucial characteristic, "excellent surgical judgment," comes through thoughtful contemplation on the results of your actions as well the actions of others.

Being "nice" is as beneficial to a physician as it is to a patient; your patients, coworkers, and other healthcare professionals all need your respect and compassion.

When faced with the decision of choosing your surgeon, I suggest, you narrow down your options by establishing a list of possible surgeons. Identify surgeons who have been approved by your insurance company or who are on the staff at the health facility you trust the most. Moreover, you can get suggestions from the doctors and nurses you encounter on a regular basis, as well as from those who have had comparable procedures.

Spending an hour on the computer digging out some potentially unpleasant information might help you avoid a disaster but the websites you choose have to be that of recognised hospitals with an excellent reputation, such as the web page of the Mayo Clinic: www.mayoclinic.org

You need to know about a surgeon's background and skill level. After you have trimmed down your list of possible surgeons, make an appointment for them to evaluate your case and for you to evaluate them. Ask if it is possible to achieve the same result using minimally invasive surgery? Through tiny incisions, many routine procedures may now be performed laparoscopically.

There are several advantages: reduced pain, faster healing, fewer infections, shorter hospital stays, and fewer medications. However, because some surgeons are not educated or trained in these approaches, they may not inform the patients about these procedures. Inquire from your doctor about how often he or she has performed this procedure and whether they specialise in it.

Surgeons develop skills and are more able to cope with difficulties when they perform specific procedures on a regular and frequent basis. According to 2009 research, the chance of major complications from the most popular kind of gastric bypass surgery decreased by 10% for every extra 10 cases performed each year by the surgeon. For novel, unusual, or difficult operations, volume is especially critical.

According to a Dartmouth College research study, the yearly

mortality rate in pancreatic cancer patients treated by surgeons who did the fewest operations was roughly four times higher than that in patients treated by surgeons who performed the highest number of operations. Here lies the problem in countries like India where the referral practice is not that robust.

The reason why few centres become centers of excellence for a particular surgery or organ in India is, there are no specific guidelines as to which surgeon is authorised to perform which surgery. The result is that many surgeons would see wonderful surgeries being performed in the conferences by experts and are willing to perform these on the first patient who comes for a consultation for that particular problem resulting in complications.

The result: the procedure gets a bad name.

Inquire about the difficulties they have experienced: good surgeons are open to discussing their poor results. It is not a reflection of failure, but rather reality, and an honest issue that demands an honest answer.

Inquire about your dangers: doctors must properly tell patients about possible risks so that they can make an informed decision, especially if the operation is elective means which are not emergencies. Go somewhere else if they can reduce the risks. Get a second opinion, if possible. If you are going to undergo a difficult or novel surgery, getting a second opinion is very vital. Check to see if there are any centres of excellence in the area. Well, it is true that not every surgeon is Dr. House, and it is true Dr. House did not become the excellent surgeon as he is portrayed in 'reel' life at one go, and even in fiction, patients had their doubts. Be it Dr. House, Dr. Thackery, or your next-door surgeon, you must ask questions to demystify the world of surgeons relating it to your complications. It is quite simple to explain what constitutes a successful lawyer, architect, or writer in a few words by stating that it is the one who wins challenging trials, constructs the greatest structures, or writes riveting novels, respectively—no other attributes would be required.

Determining what constitutes a good doctor, on the other hand, is a challenging undertaking. Because recovery is not uniform in all patients due to the simple fact that all patients and their bodies are different and react differently to stress and surgery. A good doctor is not the one who cures the most.

It is not the person who makes the best diagnosis, because, in many situations of self-limiting or incurable illnesses, an accurate and early diagnosis makes little difference to the patient.

It is not the person who understands more scientific information, because medical science is still ignorant about a lot of ailments. A good surgeon is one who knows when not to operate!

Other professions can be rated on their final outcomes, but a doctor can only be considered good if he or she possesses as many of the following characteristics as feasible. A good doctor is intelligent, honest, kind, modest, energetic, optimistic, and efficient—all at the same time. He or she instills complete trust in patients and renews the magical relationship on a regular basis, which is sufficient treatment for any condition and the finest beginning point for dealing with all causes of pain and suffering.

Although it is unusual to find so many attributes in a single person, the medical profession offers fertile ground for discovering such a combination of qualities. Fortunately, skilled doctors exist, but whether passion toward the profession is the cause of excellence remains to be seen. You just have to discover the reason for the passion and find the right doctor for you!

# 2
# BROKEN TRUST

*"Nothing is as important as passion. No matter what you want to do with your life, be passionate."* – Bon Jovi

A rolling stone collects no moss: This is a well-known proverb that portrays the fact that a frivolous person achieves nothing in life. To perfect a job path, one must settle down in life and focus on it. A person cannot be competent in all the jobs at the same time. Well, is your surgeon a well-settled person in the field, or is he a 'Jack of all trades and master of none?' The idea of surgical competence and its growth has been the subject of growing investigation.

It is a fascinating issue, and gaining a better knowledge of it will assist in advancing professional standards and patient care quality. As surgeons face increased pressure from financial cuts, larger caseloads, and longer workweeks, the desire to raise the level of knowledge has become a top priority for every forward-thinking professional. While the belief that intrinsic talent is necessary for surgical competence persists, surgeons are increasingly acknowledging the need for excellent training, even if surgeons with innate abilities may be able to train more rapidly and effectively.

It is critical to recognize that the contemporary surgeon requires a diversified skill set in order to enhance patient outcomes and care quality. Modern surgical education takes a comprehensive approach.

Its goal is to develop surgeons with the necessary technical and non-technical abilities, and maintaining this balance is crucial. When determining skill, professionalism, and the ability to engage and communicate effectively with others and manage other members of a multi-professional surgical team, must be taken into account (i.e., team player). These attributes are crucial to the success of surgical treatment.

Only a few surgeons are born, a few get trained to conduct surgery, and a few have surgery thrust on them!

This phrase is filled with so much truth! I have seen a lot of surgeons who had no idea why they became doctors. They are completely out of place in the world of surgeons and have no idea what else to do. Perhaps there was a lot of glamour linked to surgery and doctors, or perhaps there was one doctor whom they idolized. Perhaps some of their family members were surgeons who made it appear extremely simple, or perhaps there was simply no branch available that matched their rank! So, what are the qualities you would seek in a surgeon to be impressed enough to give your bodies in their hands?

My tenure as a Visiting Faculty in 2005 at the Mayo Clinic, Rochester, Minnesota, USA, was filled with extraordinary experiences. They rank as one of the best hospitals in the world. This is not merely due to the excellent infrastructure and faculty of the medical school which is awe-inspiring, but also because the care for minute details in everything that meets the eye makes it so.

Whether you are having surgery or merely getting a checkup, the doctor's bedside demeanor at the hospital is so personal and full of concern.

Most of the consultants I worked with showed excellent taste in dressing, which was very elegant but not flamboyant. It is a known fact that the doctor's response to a patient's worries and queries can significantly influence their health.

Every student that passes out from the institute developed 'patience' as a virtue and it is emphasised that if one dismisses the patient's concerns regularly, they will be less inclined to bring up future issues. All the surgeons I worked with would take the time to politely and thoroughly answer all the inquiries.

In India, most surgeons want to take a cautious approach to their patients' illnesses with the limited resources that they are provided.

With the sword of consumer courts hanging over their heads, defensive medication has become a norm rather than an exception. Over-treatment is a red flag since it implies that your surgeon may be unsure of their diagnosis. It might also indicate a concern for malpractice claims stemming from previous events. While it is human to make a mistake, an unorganized or careless doctor raises the danger of patient disease or damage.

Not only untrained doctors or surgeons but a lot of quacks and alternate medicine professionals provide care to the patients in the Indian hinterland. There was an incident in Delhi in an illegal clinic where a quack tried to operate on a patient with a shaving blade and when the patient started to bleed profusely, he abandoned the place and ran. Later the patient staggered out of the clinic into the street and died while being shifted to another hospital. It remains a fact that even the supposedly adequately trained surgeons have made blunders that are not even mentioned in the textbooks! Those are the 'never events' of the procedure. I have heard of surgeons who attempted an appendicectomy twice and ended up removing something else the first time. I also know of a few surgeons, who, after removing a gallbladder, failed to recognize the gall bladder and instead removed the intestines. The tales of such misadventures of doctors linger for days in the medical grapevine. Frequently, the patient is given a fair explanation, and the patient has no reason to question a surgeon working at a prestigious corporate hospital.

A media report outlining the agony of Bilal, a ten-year-old kid who lost his foot after being forced to shuttle from one huge hospital in Delhi to another for treatment of a foot ailment, has been taken Suo Motu by the National Human Rights Commission.

To preserve his life from infection, his foot had to be amputated. A glass piece had been missed on the initial examination and the wound turned bad. Following that, his family members transported him to a Meerut hospital, where his foot was amputated to save his life.

On January 19, 2018, the Deccan Chronicle reported a startling complaint filed by the Coimbatore City Police. Three physicians from a private hospital in Coimbatore were accused of leaving cotton and gauze pieces inside the body of a four-year-old child following kidney surgery.

Usually, complex surgeries like this have sometimes almost 15 people involved in the operation theater itself. The final swab count in these cases has to be done by the head nurse along with the doctors involved in the procedure. But the responsibility for such an unlikely event rest solely on the shoulders of the main operating surgeon who may have even left the theater by the time the wound of the patient is sutured closed to tend to other patients, leaving the responsibility of the counting process with the assistant surgeon.

I am in no way defending the surgeon who is responsible for the event, but what I want to emphasize is that India is a big country with a huge population, and extrapolation of the same guiding principles as those in the West would be out of place. In such situations, the responsibility should be shared by the other theater staff too instead of just one person being blamed and the compensation fixed according to the fee paid by the patient to the surgeon/Hospital.

Usually, the hospitals also have an equal share in the payout to the patients but the loss of the reputation of an otherwise trained surgeon is unfathomable.

Usually, the surgeon concerned would have had one complication out of the 100 cases he does, which is within the acceptable limit. Again, the patient feels that the whole amount paid to the hospital is the surgeon's fee. In actuality, only a small amount of the bill is the surgical fee (in most corporate hospitals, the charges are fixed between 11% to 15% of the whole bill).

The list of these unfortunate events is long and they are not easily understood by the layman; neither are these events as straightforward as the media tends to make it, widening the doctor-patient relationship gap.

The majority of the complaints are connected to medical malpractice in private hospitals and nursing homes because you only become a consumer when you pay for the services. However, it may not be inferred that these complications only happen in private hospitals. The Government hospitals and clinics provide free services and thus do not fall under the gambit of the consumer forum.

While training in the government hospitals, each and every student like me has witnessed complications of exceptional proportions! It is wrong to presume that when a business angle is involved, dishonesty and a negligent attitude are more likely, resulting in people suffering. A WHO-funded study estimated that 234.2 million major surgeries are performed worldwide (2008), and 3 percent to 16 percent of these would land in a complication. It was estimated that 50 percent of these complications would be preventable and 0.4%-0.8% would lead to permanent disability or death.

Now, this data is from the developed countries where the care is exceptional. The figures may be higher or lower depending upon the documentation and availability of surgical care in developing countries.

To tell you the truth, medical science is not an exact science and 4+4 may not be always 8! The WHO's figures only include nations with a medium or low economic status (which account for 80% of the worldwide population). Therefore, the true figure might be significantly higher, given that one out of every ten patients in rich countries is a victim of medical errors. These mistakes can include using pharmaceuticals in ways they were not intended to be used, making mistakes with blood transfusions and X-rays, or, in more serious circumstances, amputation of the incorrect limb or operating on the wrong side of the brain.

The lack of a defined hierarchy in certain hospitals and poor communication among the medical personnel are two reasons that contribute to such blunders. Mistakes connected to erroneous pharmaceutical prescriptions alone cost healthcare systems throughout the world $42 billion, according to the Geneva-based group (37 billion euros). Overall, the risks associated with an unneeded operation are widespread, and the cost of healthcare is high. Women are particularly vulnerable to needless surgery, with hysterectomies and cesarean sections among the most commonly overprescribed procedures.

In 2005, almost 750,000 hysterectomies were performed each year, with a stunning 90 percent of them being unnecessary (according to Goldberg in Alternative Medicine). One of the most common and unneeded procedures performed in the United States is the removal of a woman's uterus.

It is not that the patients are the only ones who suffer when something like this happens; the entire surgical community suffers as well, eroding the patient's faith in his doctor and vice versa. Patients who suffer at the hands of inexperienced and irresponsible surgeons sometimes doubt the real ones, perpetuating the vicious circle. Good surgeons now fall prey to patients whose minds are already webbed with doubts and who attack the doctors and nurses out of anxiety and lack of trust.

The attacks vary from mobs vandalizing hospital facilities and setting an ambulance on fire to physical assaults and verbal abuse by patients' attendants against physicians, nurses, and anybody wearing the white coat.

Across India, there have been reports of violence against surgeons, nurses, and paramedical employees. In June, a young doctor in Andhra Pradesh was assaulted by a gang of 12 men after performing a postmortem on their deceased relative. In the vast majority of instances, the assaults occur immediately after the physicians inform the attendants about the death of the patient. India is not the only country where medical professionals are subjected to violence; it is now a worldwide occurrence.

Between 1980 and 1990, approximately 100 healthcare professionals in the United States died as a consequence of violence. As shown in a study of 170 university hospitals, 57 percent of emergency room staff had been threatened with a weapon in the five years before the poll.

According to a study of 600 doctors by the British Medical Association in 2008, one-third of those polled had been the victim of a verbal or physical attack in the preceding year, albeit more than half of those polled (52%) did not disclose it. In China, doctors are regularly attacked. In June 2010, the son of a patient who died 13 years earlier of liver cancer viciously attacked a doctor and a nurse in Shandong province.

According to an editorial in The Lancet, the extent, regularity, and ferocity of attacks have startled the globe, with a third of doctors having been involved in war and thousands injured. In Israel, 70 percent of physicians and 90 percent of support workers working in a hospital emergency department reported violent acts, the majority of which were verbal abuse. Violence has been documented in Bangladesh, primarily in hospitals but also in private healthcare facilities. A study of 675 physicians in training from nine tertiary institutions throughout Pakistan found that 76 percent had experienced verbal or physical abuse in the previous two months.

The rise in violence against medical personnel can be attributed to a number of factors, including a general increase in social animosity, as seen by incidents of road rage and other forms of violence at schools and colleges across India.

Doctors have long been held in high respect in India mainly owing to their public image. Surgeons are often accused of malpractice due to the current perception among the people that those in the private healthcare industry are only business-minded.

Sensationalizing every news event in media, frequently neglecting to mention the facts, glossing over banal aspects, and exonerating a doctor in an incidence of alleged medical malpractice are some elements that contribute to this unfavorable image of surgeons.

Many years ago, I had a stab wound patient who was a young lad who had just refused to give the attackers his phone. He had lost a lot of blood and arrived at our emergency room at midnight on my call day. It was a little cut on the upper abdomen that was bleeding profusely.

My colleague and I examined him and discovered that the knife had pierced his stomach and rested on the pancreas, just missing a major vessel before shearing off one of the smaller branches.

We clamped the bleeder and closed the stomach perforation, and by the time we were done, it was 3 a.m., and the entire crew was exhausted. Expecting thanks from the family who had gathered outside my OR, I proudly stepped out and informed them that their kid had been rescued and that no organs had to be resected. There were no words of gratitude or thankfulness that were spoken, instead, only stillness, until an aunt asked shrilly, "How big is the wound you gave him?" I informed them that we do not usually measure the incision, but it may be roughly 10 cm to 12 cm long because I had to look at the entire abdomen. What followed was something that no one could have predicted! "Everyone is correct about you!" she said. "You guys are liars; the thug gave him a 2 cm cut, and you gave him a 12 cm cut". In the crowd's eyes, there were no thanks, only accusations.

I am normally a calm surgeon, but I could not seem to keep my emotions in check at that point in time. I was enraged, fatigued, and frustrated! I simply turned away from them! It was the only rational option I had. After a long time, the rest of the relatives, with the exception of the belligerent aunt, came to my chamber and apologized! By that time, I was already having self-doubts and devising protective methods. The fissures could already be seen. Satyamev Jayate's episode on doctors did not do much to help and heal the relations between patients and doctors. They saw me once after the boy was discharged, but it was the last time they saw me. I am guessing they saw the same things in me, the mistrust. The ultimate casualty is patient care, and most doctors begin to practice defensive medicine as a result of such instances.

There is more to surgery than can be explained by the present effort for randomized controlled trials, and other research aiming at pure science and understanding. The art and philosophy of surgery are sometimes disregarded since they are more difficult to define, teach, and maybe pass on to future generations of surgeons through formal education. Although humanism, surgical essence, and surgeon traits are rarely mentioned anymore, they are just as crucial for educating and sustaining competent surgeons.

Many surgeons, at some point in their careers, strive to define what it means to be a good surgeon. In this regard, we will try to analyze:

- the key prerequisites of becoming a good surgeon
- the attributes such a specialist should possess, based on a chosen literature research and personal experience.

The characteristics of a competent surgeon are inherently subjective, and their meanings may vary depending on whether the phrase is employed by professional colleagues, patients, and their families, or social media. Even an Internet search for the words "good surgeon" yields no quick results.

Without a doubt, a surgeon's ability to be a good surgeon is impacted by his or her education and training (which is becoming increasingly common). Two key goals should be achieved through education and training.

The first is to improve one's manual dexterity. After all, the most important aspect of a surgeon's job is manual labor. Regardless of how significant other factors may appear, a surgeon who lacks appropriate manual skills is not a surgeon.

The second goal is to get a broad range of clinical and scientific expertise in the specialty of choice. In real life, one frequently encounters surgeons who have excelled in one of these areas but not the other. Theoretical and scientific components of brilliant technicians might be absent to some extent. The urge to gain broad theoretical knowledge on complicated medical topics, on the other hand, frequently coexists with subpar performance in the operating room.

During my postgraduation days, one of my teachers and an intricate surgeon used to lecture us on how to have a successful practice after our training is over. His 'mantra' for good training was based on three principles:

A. Availability
B. Behavior
C. Competence

The idea that competence was at the bottom of his list always interested me!

Being the only urologist did not make him complacent, and he would always be accessible in his OPD at the scheduled times. He stated he would be available day after day until he retired and beyond. This is difficult to comprehend at first but it may be understood by the fact that every patient could locate him in the same spot at the same time even after many years. However, this was before the Internet!

Since then, things have evolved, and surgeons' schedules are now available in a dynamic form and even virtually. But what is the use of a doctor who is not available when the patient requires his assistance? Surgeons, even so!

The solitary factor that may make or ruin a relationship is behavior. I saw an essay a long time ago in which the author simply advised doctors to get off their 'high horses' and meet the patient where he was, at the ground level. It is no longer acceptable to just adopt a "know it all" attitude and expect patients to trust you!

It is no longer appropriate to have hurried discussions, interrupt patients in the middle of a conversation, or be impatient as other patients wait outside your outpatient facility. All scars will heal in the end!

Patients have no idea about the delicate tissue handling that a surgeon does during surgery. This rated quite high in our poll of patients when we asked about the quality one considers when making a surgical decision, which was surprising, given the fact that the inside of an operating room is never available to patients or families!

A few surgeons provide surgical films to their patients, but the face of the surgeon is never seen, and there is no way of knowing if the same surgeon operated on him or if it was an outsourced talent. Surgical competency and its appraisal combined is one of the profession's most contentious issues.

The surgical profession is grappling with the complex issue of how surgery as a specialty craft should be taught and how to assess when an individual is competent within their chosen sphere and how that competence should be maintained in the current climate of reduced working hours and shorter training.

Now, are you the passionate surgeon experienced by age or by practice? We will see next.

# 3
# EXPERIENCE MATTERS?

*"Always choose a surgeon who has white hair and piles. The white hair will make him look experienced and the piles will give him a concerned look."* – Anonymous

So, what exactly are the factors you would consider in your surgeon to give you that glitter in your eye? Age and experience? Although recent research suggests that physician age is negatively associated with clinical performance in primary care, no comprehensive research has been done on the association between surgeon age and patient outcomes. Recently, primary care research has found a negative correlation between the surgeon's age and clinical performance.

Older doctors are less likely to adopt innovative treatment procedures and provide suitable drugs. When compared to their younger colleagues, elderly physicians score worse on recertification exams and are less likely to have up-to-date knowledge. As a result of these findings, professional organizations have been urged to implement more stringent mechanisms for performance evaluation and certification throughout a physician's career.

The relationship between physician age and surgical performance is not well understood. As opposed to primary care, the surgical practice may bring unique obstacles for the older physician. Complex operations take a long time and need a lot of physical and mental energy. The previous study has shown that physical dexterity, strength, and visuospatial ability, as well as cognitive capabilities and the capacity to maintain attention, all decline with age. However, it has not been shown if such variables lead to poor patient outcomes. Two studies have found that older surgeons with coronary artery bypass grafting and carotid endarterectomy had higher fatality rates. In contrast, other studies have found that the surgeon's youth and inexperience are more relevant risk factors.

However, it has been reported that surgeons in the age group 41 to 60 years demonstrated lower mortality in their patients than that seen in patients of surgeons who were over 60 years of age in the three categories where there was a statistically significant difference—coronary artery bypass, pancreatectomy, and carotid endarterectomy. Several additional research has come to the same conclusion: surgeons' quality of work deteriorates slowly but noticeably as they become older. It is vital to remember that research involving thousands of doctors does not reveal anything about a single doctor's abilities. In the research, several elderly surgeons outperformed their younger counterparts. The results also revealed that senior surgeons who had a full workload rather than retiring into semiretirement and seeing only a few patients each week lost no expertise. It is easy to blame the drop in performance among older surgeons on the lack of fine-motor control, and this is probably true. The procedures that revealed the biggest difference between elderly and young surgeons, as the authors of the University of Michigan study pointed out, needed a high degree of cooperation. The above data may be biased and may not tell all; according to a recent review of data from over one million operations, the more procedures surgeons undertake, the better their patients' results are, at least until they reach a learning plateau, which will improve as the surgeon gains experience and gets older.

Many researchers have recognized that a surgeon's experience is connected to his or her performance over the past two decades or more, but studies in the field have been inconsistent.

Thus, there have not been many practical suggestions based on learning curve data. These are the findings of 57 recent surgical performance studies done in 14 countries with over 17,000 surgeons and 35 distinct treatment types. The majority of studies looked at the number of patients a surgeon treated, and some also took into account the years of experience. Researchers showed that when the surgeon's number of previous cases grew, the time required for the procedure, the incidence of recurrence of the problem, complication rates, blood transfusion requirements, death rates, and stroke rates all improved. It has been said that a surgeon's performance might degrade at the end of his or her career. During a 20-year study, older surgeons who operated on the thyroid gland were more likely than the others to cause recurrent laryngeal nerve injury and hypoparathyroidism, both of which are associated with significant consequences. Before electing to have surgery, patients have the right to know how good the surgeon or the surgical team is. They should have access to statistics on individual team outcomes. These results will be better for more experienced surgeons, according to this recent evaluation of the evidence. However, performance escarpments after a period demonstrate the necessity to maintain the data up to date in order to keep doctors on their toes. In general, the most experienced surgeons may be found in big, centralized hospitals with specialized centers. Patients may also want to learn about the overt risk-related indicators, such as anticipated complication rates, in addition to a surgeon's expertise in performing a certain surgery. Patients may also want to consider a variety of quality metrics at the hospital where the surgery is being conducted, such as whether a specialist unit or dedicated operating room exists for a specific kind of treatment, as well as how many of such procedures have been performed there.

Patients should also take into account a surgeon's ability to communicate and create a trusting connection.

When I initially started my career as a surgeon, I had no idea of the areas where I lacked adequate knowledge. I also made mistakes and learned by trial and error about how to improve my methods, such as how to monitor a patient's safety and anticipate and respond to any problems that develop. Similarly, years of surgical experience have taught me how to spot a patient in distress so that I can intervene swiftly and correctly. On one of my evening rounds, I found one of my patients restless. It was the 2nd postoperative day and the 1st day was uneventful. The nurses had started the patient on a soft diet as usual (as per the post-op order).

This patient, however, had chronic obstructive pulmonary disease (COPD) and had difficulty breathing. To add to that, he developed slow gastric emptying and sluggish intestine (common in the post-op period in intestinal surgery; called paralytic ileus). Together, the situation produced a drop in oxygen levels and irritability. A hand on the abdomen was all that was required. We shifted the patient to the ICU and juggled with the oral fluids and oxygen supplementation, which was all that was required. If I had missed his symptoms, he would not have made it through the night!

Every successful surgeon has tons of these stories to tell. Experienced surgeons are the ones who contribute to research in the particular field, develop new ways based on their knowledge, and share their knowledge with peers and students who wish to improve their skills.

Furthermore, experienced workers are frequently aware of several approaches to achieving a goal. They can provide you with treatment alternatives and they know how to adapt their method to reach the greatest potential outcome in a variety of conditions.

They have more tools in their toolkit, so to speak, which is to a patient's benefit when undergoing a surgical operation because they stand to receive the best treatment plan personalized to them. Along with a surgeon's years of experience, the experience in one particular field gives a few surgeons an edge as well.

I know an orthopedic surgeon who now performs only joint replacement surgeries, and that too, only knee replacements!

And oh boy! He does a ton of them each month. A general plastic surgeon's outcome may differ from those of a facial plastic surgery expert, for example. Even though both doctors have 15 years of experience, a general plastic surgeon may only conduct a few facelifts per year, but a facial plastic surgery expert has a better grasp of facial operations and performs facelifts every week. In the US, the surgeon's skill in a certain specialist field is demonstrated by board certification, whereas in India, there are no such criteria. Most surgeons learn and update their skills by attending conferences, and those who can afford, learn by going abroad for an 'Observership' in their chosen field under a surgeon with a high caseload doing only that type of surgery.

One way to find out about the surgeon's expertise in a specific surgical procedure is to question the surgeon directly about the number of times he gets to perform the said procedure routinely. You can ask your surgeon whether he has undergone further training through a fellowship performed under the supervision of a more experienced surgeon. Fellowships provide surgeons with the most comprehensive training with certain sorts of treatments and further illustrate your doctor's commitment to their profession and specialty. However, it may be not needed for all surgical specialties.

Let us look at the various factors which affects the patients choice in seeking the best outcome from a surgeon.

### Age Of The Surgeon

Now the question is, amidst all the factors, is age a relevant factor for surgeons? Generally speaking, age improves a doctor's proficiency with procedures. Experience adds a lot of nuance and speed to their technique. The main limiting factor that will dull their skill is age-related tremors and/or declining strength due to poor health. Even then, they can compensate for their shortcomings by asking a younger surgeon to assist them or by mainly performing a lot of robot-assisted surgeries where the tremors and fatigue are negated by the surgeon sitting and doing the surgeries on a console, and the tremors are taken care of by the robotic arm.

The major problems that cannot be compensated are loss of mental acuity and recall and problems in cognition.

But in an active surgeon, these usually only become issues past the late 70s or early 80s and are easily perceived when they examine or interview you.

According to a new study, surgeons in their mid-career, between the ages of 35 and 60, are the safest for patients.

Newly qualified surgeons are likely to make a few( read: more than a few) errors. Surgeons are believed to attain their optimum performance after around ten years of expertise in their chosen area. However, while some surgeons cease operations as they get older, recognizing that they are no longer as nimble or observant as they once were, no one knows how long their time of excellence lasted. According to results published online by the British Medical Journal, the performance of surgeons who have been doing the same procedures for more than 20 years may begin to decrease.

Is it true that the older you are, the more experience and expertise you have? Is that correct? Wrong! The surgeon, too, has an expiry date! Typically, this is what distinguishes surgeons from physicians. Physical fitness is required of a surgeon. It is a life-or-death situation! A young surgeon may be inexperienced and eager to take on assignments that are above his or her pay grade. A senior surgeon may have a lot of expertise and leave a lot to a rookie surgeon, or he or she may not be able to complete the entire surgical process.

The difficulty is to find a balance in our pursuit of the perfect blend. Surgical performance is a reflection of more than just technical abilities. Experience, cognitive abilities, dexterity, visuospatial ability, and environmental variables all contribute to the capacity to do a task effectively, methodically, and safely. In a recent piece headlined "When is a surgeon too old to operate?" the New York Times explored this issue. They talked about an 80-year-old Chief of Vascular Surgery at a New Jersey hospital who was the first doctor to be reviewed by a new aging surgeon program, which found that "he could capably continue operating" after testing.

"Approximately one-third of all practicing surgeons are beyond the age of 55," according to the American College of Surgeons.

When I get into the boots of a patient looking for the right surgeon for my procedure, I would look at the whole picture, rather than the age of the surgeon alone. It is like an Indian arranged marriage. You get married to the whole family rather than to just the bride or the bridegroom! So, we should look at the surgeons who have a vibrant team headed by an older surgeon. The team should have a healthy mix of young ones and the older, more experienced surgeons who would together do their best to save you in the worst-case scenarios.

## Personality/Demeanor

So many times, in my job, I have seen the patients' delight when they meet a well-dressed doctor, they can call their own! We are drawn to powerful physiques and attractive appearances because we feel comfortable with the person who looks after us. In the past, the witch doctors were the only ones in with a hamlet, but that is no longer the case.

When looking for the appropriate individual for their procedure, people have a lot of choices, and your looks and personality make a difference. People look at the surgeons as a package. In addition to your personality, patients look at the car you drive, the watch you wear, and the phone you are holding. This is not just hearsay, but I can tell you this from personal experience.

A patient told me that he would not entrust his life in the hands of a surgeon who had a cracked phone screen! Really? He said anyone who cannot take care of his phone can hardly take care of his patients! On probing further, he told me that everyone would be considered capable in a big hospital like ours because the bad apples would not be able to survive the competition. But he would like to know how successful a doctor, his surgeon is and he would find that by how the surgeon presents himself. A successful surgeon would be dressed powerfully and exudate confidence.

Well, all patients may not agree with him, but to a certain extent, it makes sense. How can a surgeon who makes a living treating diabetic foot and abscess afford a BMW?

## Compassion and Empathy

A doctor must be an excellent listener as well as a speaker. A surgeon more so. A successful surgeon understands that the practice of medicine is reliant on the exchange of ideas, concepts, and orders. Incorrect information might cause major issues.

To deduce signals from a patient's body language, a doctor needs be adept in both verbal and nonverbal communication. Also, because a doctor needs to deal with patients, their families, and his staff on a regular basis, using the appropriate tone, idioms, and vocabulary is an important part of the medical profession.

I had anger issues! And as a surgeon, I always wanted to be in command at all times. More so because I realized that to repeatedly get the same results we needed to replicate the same steps all the time. That is the right way, except I did not effectively communicate what I wanted the people around me to understand and respond. I would just yell at them when things were not going the way I had wanted it to go. It was like a child who wanted ice cream, but when he did not get it, he resorted to wailing at the top of his voice! Did it help? To a certain extent, people were afraid and I could bulldoze my way through getting my work done. But then I realized that this behavior of mine made the environment around me tense, and the assisting nurse was dropping important instruments just because she was so tense. The assistant surgeons would end up holding the camera too tightly reducing the manoeuvrability of the instruments, and more so, I was dead tired by the end of the procedures. I seemed to age faster, and after every major surgery, the results were good but I felt like I gave a part of myself away and felt reduced in size. After 30 years of surgical practice, I now recognize that there are other ways, more efficient ways to get the work done without losing a piece of oneself.

Empathy solves most of my problems now without losing life

and limb. The nurses have their own problems. If instruments are malfunctioning, someone up the ladder does not care; so, what is the point in telling the nurse?

If he patient was very sick and I tried my best but could not save him. Not my fault and empathy for oneself is the best thing that you can give yourself. We are not Gods and should not try to become one! I am much happier now. People like to work with me and patients come to me for surgeries and friends entrust me with their patients and parents, especially the ones they are very fond of. I am happy to claim that I am a no-frills surgeon. If you need to get the work done, send your patient to me!

We all recognize that a surgeon is not a machine that is programmed to execute a task. A doctor's personality includes empathy, compassion, kindness, and politeness. Patients respond better to a doctor who understands their requirements. As a result, a doctor's focus should be on treating patients with civility and compassion. When dealing with patients, presence and patience are essential. Understanding the patient's concerns requires mental presence. Instead of worrying about how to reply, a doctor should focus on what the patient is saying (verbal and nonverbal indications). Like the wellness coach Graham Green puts it, "when we want to engage with someone, put the person first and tell yourself that he is more important and just listen to him. It is fascinating, how much you can learn from the people's stories".

A doctor's patience is tested when it comes to being present in the moment and focusing all of one's attention on the patient. It is important to recognize that merely wearing a white coat does not automatically confer respect; rather, respect must be earned. A patient is less likely to seek care from another physician if he is happy and does not feel neglected.

If you want to be a doctor, you must develop professional abilities and maintain a professional demeanour. Working with human life may be quite stressful, and a doctor must be emotionally strong to cope with these stressors on a regular basis.

An emotionally stable individual can effectively manage

emergency situations and human suffering.

He should also be up to speed on all current developments and medical news. A doctor should be eager to learn new technologies and increase his knowledge and abilities through training. He should be able to design techniques fast and use appropriate data. Respect for others is something that cannot be taught; it has to come from within.

While we all desire excellent medical treatment, we also want physicians who listen to us and have empathy and understanding for our thoughts and worries expressed via a kind approach.

This can assist us in developing trust and a sense of connection with them. However, such a mixture might be difficult to come by. Only 53 percent of 800 recently hospitalized patients believed their doctors were sympathetic and compassionate, according to a 2011 poll. These figures might actually reflect reality and not just be a figment of the patients' imagination.

Researchers discovered that clinicians frequently disregarded or rejected matters of concern indicated by patients, delivering empathetic reactions just 22 percent of the time in one study where doctor-patient meetings were filmed. Similar findings have been seen in other investigations. Following a flood of studies pointing to the far-reaching advantages of emotionally attentive surgeons, thought leaders have been looking into methods to bring greater empathy into the medical industry. That means rethinking who should be admitted to medical school in the first place, as well as what they should learn while they are there.

According to recent studies, patients who have doctors who listen to them and show that they understand their concerns follow their doctors' orders more closely, are more satisfied with their treatment, and have better health; for example, they recover from colds faster and show physiological signs of a stronger immune system. Patients who thought their surgeons were very compassionate during their hospital stay, were 20 times more likely to think their procedure went well.

Furthermore, research shows that physicians with greater

empathy levels—that is, those who are aware of their patient's emotional needs and respond properly to them—experience less stress, cynicism, and burnout than those with lower empathy levels did. Several studies have found a link between physicians' cognitive empathy and better patient outcomes, including one in which diabetic patients with high cognitive empathy had better management of their condition and fewer diabetes-related problems needing hospitalization.

Sophie Johnson has this to say in her article on the Qualities of a Surgeon in CHRON: Surgeons must like learning since it is a lifetime commitment and one of the most crucial qualities of a surgeon is to stay current with new medical information.

Mental acuity in specific areas, particularly memory and recall, is required to obtain the necessary surgical knowledge. In diagnosis and treatment planning, recalling knowledge about the body, its ailments, and prospective therapies is critical.

One of the abilities required for a surgeon to properly treat patients is the problem-solving ability, which includes the capacity to think on one's feet. Being meticulous and attentive aids a surgeon in keeping track of all aspects of a patient's treatment. Because no two days are the same, surgeons must love diversity and unpredictability. Empathy enables the doctor to communicate with patients and assess their well-being. Because patients are not always at their best, patience and professionalism are frequently required. Patience in problem-solving and weighing the pros and cons of the different treatment options can lead to enhanced medical knowledge and sound surgical judgment.

The impact of surgeon experience on perioperative and postoperative outcomes has been studied extensively. Experience is clearly vital in several sectors, such as administration, finance, and engineering. But how can we effectively assess a surgeon's experience? There is no set way to go about it.

The degree of expertise and the number of surgeries performed per year are used to define a surgeon's experience in lung cancer therapy in the medical literature. Furthermore, the research implies that to be qualified to do an operation alone, it is essential to have performed a minimum number of surgeries aided by a senior surgeon.

However, it is true that your surgeon's experience cannot be measured by the number of years he has worked or his age. It is the proficiency, the passion, and the ethics followed by the surgeon that makes him the superior kind. What is your doctor's inspiration? Let us find his 'IKIGAI.'

# 4
# I LOVE MY IKIGAI

*"Retire to the center of being, which is calmness!"* -Paramahansa Yogananda

Ikigai (ee-key-guy) is a Japanese notion that combines the phrases iki and gai, which indicate 'alive' or 'life,' and 'benefit' or 'value,' respectively. When these phrases are used together, they refer to what gives your life value, meaning, or purpose. Ikigai is a Japanese concept that is related to the French term 'raison d'etre,' which means 'cause for being.'

The notion of Ikigai is thought to have originated from traditional Japanese medicine's core health and wellness concepts. This medical tradition maintains that one's mental-emotional health and sense of purpose in life have an impact on one's physical well-being. A surgeon's IKIGAI will give you the best results when you want to undergo an operation! That one procedure, that one branch, that one surgery that he is so good at and passionate about, is the one that he takes to the next level and gives the patient the best clinical outcome.

According to the Japanese psychologist Michiko Kumano (2017), Ikigai is a feeling of happiness that emerges from a commitment to activities that one appreciates and is associated with a sense of completion.

Michiko goes on to separate Ikigai from fleeting pleasure (hedonia in the old Greek meaning) and match it with eudaimonia, the ancient Greek concept of a well-lived life that leads to the best and most permanent type of happiness. Gai is the key to discovering the significance or meaning of your life.

The Ikigai Venn diagram, which depicts the overlapping of the four primary qualities—what you are excellent at, what the world needs, what you can be paid for, and, of course, what you love—is the greatest method to absorb the underlying idea of Ikigai truly. If you bring it down to its most basic principle, Ikigai exists at the intersection of these points. The Ikigai of a person is highly personal; it is a mental condition that allows one to feel at peace and gives life a purpose. The existence of Ikigai is associated with a low level of stress and a general sense of well-being. Okinawans (Japanese people from the East China Sea islands) who follow Ikigai are among the world's longest-living people.)

Throughout our medical careers, we frequently look for solutions to the following questions:

- What am I hoping to accomplish?
- Which procedure is becoming popular among patients and surgeons?
- What areas of specialization or sub-specialization would I wish to pursue?
- What is it that I want to do when I am a consultant?
- What is the value creation I will achieve when I get trained in a particular procedure?
- Will I be able to make enough or will I just make a living?
- How much pleasure or satisfaction will I achieve in practicing a particular branch or procedure?

Ikigai means different things to different surgeons. For an average surgeon, his Ikigai connections occur at a very late stage, when he is going into one of the specialties of his choosing. In fact, by the conclusion of the MBBS and internship, most of the doctors would have no idea about what they want to become!

Some doctors choose their specialization after MBBS based on the experiences of their seniors, but later branch out into a different field. A few of them would choose a specialty, purely based on how much revenue they could earn after their training is over. Some of them would have chosen a certain specialization based on the fact that either of their parents or someone else in the family was into the same branch or profession.

Hence, moving in the same direction would be easier as they would concentrate on that particular field, and eventually, as qualified surgeons, they would be more readily incorporated into the profession that their father or mother had built up over the years.

But many doctors, including myself, have no idea about their specialized path. Throughout my MBBS program, I aspired to be a physician. 1 could never imagine myself as a surgeon, even if I thought I would like to become one. Unfortunately, because there were so many lockdowns throughout my internship, we could not work in the wards as clinicians and pick which department we wanted. The options were quite restricted at the time. The number of seats available for each specialty was extremely restricted, with only eight seats available in each medical college in surgery and there were only five of them in Rajasthan.

We had to sit for an examination (like the present-day NEET, but with much tougher competition), after which we would be granted a seat based on merit. It seemed as though God had hand-picked something for me. I wanted to be a physician, but I missed out on a seat by one mark.

The final medicine (Physician) seat was taken by the person just ahead of me on the merit list and I was devastated. I was left with the option of General Surgery.

And thus began my profession in surgery in the wards of Udaipur where there were a lot of Urology patients (my boss was a urologist of repute) and I would carry the smell of urine on me to my mess and beyond. There were a variety of general surgery patients there, as well as burns victims. Then there were the head trauma cases. The burns patients were the worst because young women would come in with suicidal or homicidal burns, which accounted for almost 95 percent of the cases.

The worst aspect about 'burns' is that no one dies right away, and people suffered a great deal over the course of many days. It seems unlikely that in certain regions of the globe where resources are plentiful, doctors are able to save burns victims with 95 percent to 100 percent burns. However, the stay of a 95 percent burns patient in our institution was practically very short as he/she would die within a week of admission. According to my seniors and experienced folks, only patients who had around 30 percent burns (body surface area) were likely to be saved. However, the anguish that would follow would be unimaginable. One would observe that these patients who were suicidal, had made a decision at the heat of the moment and thought that they would die early, but that is not the case. They would have to get admitted in the burns ward under a cage-like cover and stay for days together. The burn wound would need to be dressed day in and day out every day, and the stench after a while would make even the close relatives puke at least once a day. There would be repeated occasions when we had to take these patients into the operating room, and the next-of-kin would be pleading because they want to see them alive. They would be hopeful inside, but we all knew there was none. Each one of the burns patients who attempted suicide and survived was remorseful. The pain was simply too much to bear. Patients in these situations might suffer for hours, days, and even months. Eventually, a certain type of infection or sepsis will just take them away. It soon became clear to me that there was no glamor or attraction in those wards and nothing that would entice me to join the surgical practice.

It is when I walked into the operating room and observed that how the professor performed the surgery that I started to have a tiny bit of hope that someday you may do things the same way or slightly better. As I begin doing a tiny bit of surgery, my self-esteem, which had taken a battering the previous day, is restored to a little extent.

I cannot recall exactly when I started to think of myself as a surgeon, but after 36 years of practice, I can say that I would not have been anything if I had not been a surgeon!

## The hunt for my Ikigai

For most surgeons, the realization arrives late. For a few, never. Because for Ikigai to appear, the surgeon must first comprehend the subject, then himself, and then the market, and finally, he must feed his family. He understands that, but yes, the Ikigai that he desired is the procedure that he is skilled at, and he will likely become one of the best in the world.

It is the feeling of accomplishment you receive after successfully performing a tough procedure that most other surgeons would avoid undertaking, and getting rewarded for it. Then you see a patient's joyful face after this surgery, and you realize that, yes, this is my Ikigai.

So, any doctor who passes their NEET test, (or PRE-PG as we used to call it back in those days, our pre-postgraduate examination), has no idea what lies ahead for them. For instance, I had an incredibly brilliant classmate. Now, this gentleman, let us call him Brijesh, was quite clever, and he was always the topper in the class. And this is not a made-up narrative; it is a true story.

Brijesh had no money issues because his family's finances were quite robust. Most of us would struggle to get placed in the first 200 ranks in the merit list of the PRE-PG exam, but this gentleman entered the exam and was placed in the top three. So, most of the students who got the higher ranks would opt for either Pediatrics or Gynecology followed closely by Radiology, (which is a fantastic career option).

Radiology is unique and preferred by very intelligent young graduates as there are no significant emergencies until an unless you want to be a interventional radiologist, and it is a nine-to-five work with no pressure to get a clientele. You can have a wonderful balance between work-life and family-life, and usually, be highly compensated as well. Aware of the possibilities, Brijesh concluded that a nickel and dime practice was not for him and enrolled in Radiology. However, six months into the Radiology course, he would often say, "I don't believe I can do this. I can't actually live without interaction with the patients. I need to treat people. I just cannot give a diagnosis and let the others do the real job of treating"!

A few days later, he took up another PRE-PG examination while doing PG in Radiology and passed it with flying colors, placing him in the top ten. He took up surgery as a profession this time. But yet again it was an excruciatingly painful six months. He used to get irritated when he had to attend ward rounds or get real and dirty in surgery. He would go and talk to the radiologists and tell them how much he missed radiology and that he did not think he was cut out for surgery. And then, after talking to a lot of people, he decided to quit surgery and made up his mind about the next specialty he would try for. Money was not an issue and intelligence was not an issue either. He went on and appeared in the PRE-PG examination once more, this time for Dermatology.

Dermatology practice was fairly pleasant; it was a nine-to-five job that paid well and had a large patient base by default. He had no problems getting through again and got the dermatology option that he sought. He ended up in Dermatology, which he did not really enjoy either.

So, after 30 months of juggling between various residency programs, he picked a subject that he did not like! The sad part was that after the third attempt, he went into severe depression because he believed that one branch was superior to the other. He married because he believed that married life would make things better for him, which was never the case. He was unable to deal with the issues and was unable to resolve any of his conflicts.

So, after a two-year fight with depression, and despite having a brilliant mind and a marriage, we learned that he consumed a poison for which there was no antidote. This was after a small squabble at home. He had taken a substance called dimethyl bromide (DEB), which is used as a grain preservative. He researched and calculated the dose which was around ten times the fatal dose. He was brought to the emergency in a slightly disoriented state and he was in pain.

We went there to see him, and having spent so much time with him, it was heartbreaking to see him die like that. In the end, he repeatedly said that he did not want to die but we could not do anything for him. He was just so damn brilliant that he beat us everywhere. He left us with no choices. A wonderful life wasted!

So, if someone says, "I was born to be a surgeon," or "I was meant to be a physician," the truth is that you will never know how it feels unless you dive into the subject. Once you have completed your three-year residency program, you will be a proper clinician in whichever discipline you choose, whether it is orthopedics, gynecology, or general surgery.

So, there you have it: the fundamentals of surgical science. Some of them do not know and do not want to stop there; they want to do more. So, at that moment, they will decide that surgery is no longer for them and that they want to be a urologist, a cardiothoracic surgeon, or a neurosurgeon.

Although an MS degree would be adequate, many after receiving their master's degree (Master in Surgery), frequently continue to accumulate further degrees as they concentrate on one region of the body. Those are the super-specialty branches

After I completed my MS residency program, I appeared for many super specialty entrance examinations and continued to be rejected! While appearing and getting rejected in these examinations, I discovered minimal access surgery at Sir Ganga Ram Hospital in New Delhi. For the first time, I saw minimum access or laparoscopic surgery performed, and I said to myself, "That's my thing." I fell in love with the subject and left everything else. That has been my thing, ever since I jumped right in and started working on it.

I received praise from my boss during my first operation as a laparoscopic surgeon. I am not sure if it was simply to lift my spirits or if it was a real compliment and he felt that way, but it helped. I began to work harder in order to achieve my goal.

When I completed my registrar-ship, I felt secure enough to take things in my hand and execute procedures that other surgeons could not. I was ready for a consultant's position and was far ahead in the game compared to my peers from the same college. But God had a different idea for me and I began to dislike Delhi.

Of course, I was just a small-town boy underneath and could not handle a metro. I got married to another small-town girl in Delhi and both of us knew straight away that Delhi could be very overwhelming! We needed to return to our roots. I returned to Jaipur and tried every hospital, but could not get a job despite being one of the few well-trained laparoscopic surgeons at that time. I simply wanted to be one step ahead of everyone. I began researching other sectors such as bariatric surgery, which was just taking root in India, and then advanced hernia repair, gastric reflux procedures, and so on. However, bariatric surgery piqued my interest, and I decided to travel to the United States to study from the finest. Fortunately, I got a break from the Mayo Clinic and was offered a student exchange program.

By the time I was already a consultant here and doing major laparoscopic procedures in India. I discovered that the fellowship kindled my interest even more because of the sheer number of surgeries that were being performed in that institution and the correct methods that were being followed; the methodical approach to a patient was absolutely blissful to watch. The techniques were simple yet fantastic. There was a lot of scientific research as well, which was even more fascinating.

So, I believed I had my Ikigai at that time, and I am still thrilled when I see a bariatric patient now. I like doing the surgery. I enjoy visiting the patient after surgery, and I enjoy being compensated for my efforts. And believe me when I say that I do not compare myself to others.

But everything I do, I do it from the bottom of my heart. And I believe that is all Ikigai is about. And different folks have their own thing which they love doing. I know a surgeon who enjoys performing only bottom surgeries and feels thrilled about it, and then there is a surgeon who performs a lot of non-scalpel vasectomies with little incisions and is quite proficient at it.

It is a tiny surgery compared with a bariatric procedure but he has done tons of them and is actually so proud of his achievement. If ever I needed to undergo a vasectomy, I guess, I will get it done through him.

I have seen a number of cancer surgeons who specialize in robotic surgery for colorectal cancer and are quite good at it. That is their Ikigai. So, it would not matter to them if you paid them less at a certain point in time since they are enthusiastic about their profession. I know a surgeon who stated, "I will pay my patient because I want to perform that procedure." It saves me so much time to be on the console of a robot while performing the procedure. In other areas, if you put in more effort to get trained, you will get reimbursed more, but this is not the case in surgery. If you are an expert in a particular operation, you will attract a large number of patients, and this is how you will get rewarded.

Your remuneration would be in terms of the joy you experience when you see your patients in the OPD ( out patient department) and work them up; then, you get to the diagnosis, you take him up for surgery, and you decide everything. Next, you take the patient into the operating room, and early in the morning when you make the first incision, you know you are doing something that will bring satisfaction to not only yourself, but also to the patient and the relatives. I still get butterflies in my stomach when I do a bariatric procedure. The feeling is incredible when these patients come back to me for follow-up and tell me the stories of their lives. How a young boy now has a girlfriend, how a woman is able to take care of her daughter after a divorce, and how a girl finally gets married after losing weight and sends me her marriage invitation card! Well, I got paid too, for all these surgeries.

So, the love was an added bonus! That is what Ikigai is all about.

Surgeons do not know their Ikigai until they enter practice and begin their careers. During their careers, they define themselves and the attitudes they uncover. They discover the disease they would like to treat and then they find a mentor who is an expert in that particular field. And after learning from their mentor, they begin to do the surgery, and in certain cases, they may even outperform their mentors. It takes a huge amount of character to become a mentor. They provide us with sound guidance, personal counseling, and encouragement to help us progress. These guys are just incredible and provide insights in addition to instructions in a particular field. They not only inspire us but also leave a significant impact on our lives. Because of this profound effect, most surgeons who reach greatness have at least one mentor, if not more. Some mentors excel at the technical aspects and motivate us to do operations with competence, accuracy, and simplicity. Other mentors have exceptional interpersonal abilities. These doctors help their mentees to improve their communication skills so that they may form fruitful connections with their patients, coworkers, and teams.

Getting to the top and being the greatest is virtually always linked to excellent mentoring. That is what an Ikigai provides. Surgeons sometimes connect greatness with mastery of the surgical technique, leading to the incorrect belief that the greatest surgeon is the most skilled. Many surgeons like and respect colleagues who demonstrate technical ability and possess the abilities required to complete the most challenging phases of an operation. An operation's ultimate purpose is to assist the patient, not the surgeon. Although a skilled surgeon possesses a rare ability that, when used properly, can provide huge benefits for the patient, being the best surgeon also entails avoiding the narcissistic concept implied in the attitude "I have done what others could not," and instead focusing on whether what we have done is beneficial to the patient. We learn and train to help the ill, to cure where we can, and to alleviate what we cannot heal during our lives as physicians.

The finest surgeons are those who are always pushing themselves to perform only what is best for the patient, not just what is "possible."

Medicine is a vast subject, and it is impossible for one person to know everything there is to know about it. You are unlikely to go wrong if you select a surgeon for whom the center of his world is your condition. Of course, this does not imply that he is doing a lot of these particular procedures, but it does imply that he enjoys doing them and will put his heart and soul into them! Falling in love with a career is similar to falling in love with a person. You either feel it or you do not, and it does not always reflect poorly on the doctor. Surgery, on the other hand, is not a necessary evil for the finest surgeons. It is a decision that he has to make.

The surgeons with their Ikigai in place are fortunate enough to be able to combine work and have the pleasure too. Did you find a doctor who gave his full attention to your problem, who enjoyed seeing you, and who charged what he charges usually or even more than what others in the same field did? Was he/she concerned about your reservations and detected things in your condition that the others had missed? Believe me, he/she is your surgeon!

# 5
# CHOOSE YOUR DOCTOR

*"Trust has to be earned. You can't trust someone hiding in a closet."*
-    House, M.D., Season 2, Episode 19 House vs. God

Transparency and trust are the two most important aspects of the doctor-patient relationship. This relationship is one of the most profound and poignant experiences that humans have ever shared. This connection, as well as the experiences that result from it, is not always ideal. The doctor-patient relationship involves a voluntary connection in which the patient deliberately seeks the surgeon's aid and the physician knowingly accepts the individual as a patient.

At its most basic level, the doctor-patient relationship is a fiduciary relationship in which the physician, when entering into the relationship, agrees to respect the patient's autonomy, maintain confidentiality, explain treatment options, obtain informed consent, provide the highest standard of care, and not abandon the patient without giving him or her adequate time to find a new doctor. On the other hand, such a contractual definition fails to capture the vast and fundamental nature of the doctor-patient relationship.

Physicians are occasionally privy to secrets, anxieties, and fears that patients have not yet shared with friends or family. Patients believe that they can maintain or restore their health and well-being by putting their confidence in a doctor. They can maintain or restore their health and well-being by putting their confidence in a surgeon. Mutual knowledge, trust, loyalty, and esteem are the four main characteristics of this unique partnership.

The surgeon learns about the patient and the patient learns about the doctor and this is the knowledge we are referring to.

The patient's faith in the surgeon's competence and compassion and the doctor's faith in the patient and his or her beliefs and symptom reports are all based on trust. The readiness of a patient to forgive a doctor for any inconvenience or error and the doctor's determination not to forsake a patient is referred to as loyalty. Patients should feel that their doctor cares about them as people and is on their side. The cornerstone of the doctor-patient interaction is made up of all these aspects.

Word-of-Mouth (WOM) is the most dependable source of information a patient may have prior to making a surgical decision, especially if it comes from another patient who underwent surgery for the same condition and reported high satisfaction levels.

A patient who underwent the said surgery by a particular surgeon may not have any biases or prejudices and would be the most reliable source of information. After all, what does an ex-patient of a surgeon stand to gain by giving positive reviews of his experience as a form of gratitude for the good service provided? What is better than receiving the information from the horse's mouth? It may be a colleague or a boss or just a relative who can testify to a satisfying surgical experience under a particular surgeon for a particular procedure. I give the highest credit points to this kind of reference because there are no kickbacks involved here and no vested interest except the goodwill of the doctor and the welfare of the patient.

However, most people who move from place to place may not have the luxury of discovering and being treated by someone like that.

We have recently become more conscious of the relevance of WOM. WOM can be beneficial, resulting in new business and patient referrals. It has been found that WOM marketing is an important consideration when choosing a hospital or a surgeon. About half of those polled say they chose a new surgeon or hospital based on recommendations from friends and family. The majority of studies agree that family, friends, or coworkers have a considerable role in the choice of the hospital and the doctor.

Information travels via word of mouth, either directly (one to one) or through the Internet and social media. Of course, the overarching goal is to provide a pleasant personal experience with each interaction. And, against a backdrop of excellent service, the goal is to generate good WOM recommendations. However, in today's world, the majority of closed groups and forums will share information about the physicians who treated and cured them. WOM from a trusted source is like gold!

But I have some serious reservations about this 'e-word of mouth' (e-WOM). e-WOM is an untrustworthy source. This is a double-edged sword: the review could be in your favour if it is a genuine one, but there are reviews and likes that can be bought for a small fee! How can you put your trust in a system that has no credibility and no genuine interest in the future patient except to direct the patient's attention toward a particular doctor? These patients are really faceless and there is no way to find out the truth or reality in the virtual world.

Do not get me wrong: a lot of reviews might be genuine. However, quite a few of these reviews could be the result of the secretary of the surgeon forcing the patients to 'rate' their experience at the time of discharge from the hospital. But is it the truth and only 100 percent truth? Possibly not! We will deal with that information source later. But let us clear our minds first and imagine a scenario where you are a patient who has experienced stomach pain through the previous night.

You decide to consult your routine healthcare provider first thing the next morning!

You are asked to undergo an ultrasound of the abdomen and your healthcare provider tells you your pain is caused by the presence of stones in the gall bladder! What will you do?

You could start your search for a good surgeon based on the recommendations of your primary healthcare provider (family physician) or the doctor who advised you to undergo surgery. They might be able to assist you in finding a quality surgeon, especially if they are the ones who informed you that you require surgery. However, you must make sure you inquire, "Why are you suggesting this surgeon to me?" If the answer is "He accepts your insurance," keep looking for another surgeon; if the answer is "This is whom we chose when my family needed a surgeon," you have a good recommendation. But be careful, the system of kickbacks is florid everywhere, and like in the other systems, corruption may be present here too. The chances of your primary care physician being solely interested in the dole is very less; he may be genuinely interested in your welfare and he knows that after all, you are going to come back to him if there are repercussions in the future! Now the problem arises when he knows that three particular surgeons are all good at their work, but he insists that you go to the one he is most friendly with; this is a red flag. The next thing you would do is whip out your phone and go to Google brother for advice. It is obvious that you need more information on the subject and where else can you get it easily? The culture now is to use the internet to help us make practically all of our decisions. We used to rely on professional reviewers, but now we use reviews from Rotten Tomatoes, Yelp, TripAdvisor, and Amazon to pick what movies to watch, restaurants to visit, hotels to book, and gadgets to purchase. For better or worse, we depend on the views of regular people, who may have prejudices, little understanding of the subject, or a proclivity to overreact to minor issues. About a decade ago, the crowdsourcing concept made its way into the medical field. It is easy to understand why, given the growing healthcare expenses, perplexing insurance options, and a cultural change in which many young people prefer urgent care centres to primary care providers.

The results of studies looking into internet reviews have not been pleasant. Consider the following study from the Hospital for Special Surgery in New York: The ratings of 275 randomly chosen sports-medicine professionals on three major review sites were examined and revealed minimal correlation—a doctor may have been rated with five stars on one site and two stars on another.

According to sports-medicine surgeon Anil Ranawat, MD, principal author of the study and associate professor at the Hospital for Spinal Surgery, if patients choose their physician entirely based on Internet reviews and their insurance, there is a strong chance they will not be happy. On one review site, a patient gave a one-star rating to a five-star obstetrician-gynecologist in Assam after waiting for weeks for the appointment and then finally getting a call from a staff member the week before notifying her that her appointment had been canceled and she would have to reschedule. While the patient found the condition frustrating, a review like this does not indicate the doctor's true level of care. And if a consultant MD just has a few reviews, a negative review like this might make a significant impact on her total rating. Doctors who are younger, get much higher evaluations than those who are older. Of course, this might indicate a more modern approach to patient care, but it is also possible that younger doctors are more Internet savvy. Many Internet rating systems may be falsified, as numerous organizations that assist doctors in improving their rankings have discovered.

Another issue is that patients frequently lack the medical knowledge necessary to evaluate a doctor's performance. A well-recognized study undertaken at the Cedars-Sinai Medical Center in Los Angeles revealed no link between how patients rated staff surgeons and their results-driven performance measures. Even with excellent performance statistics (successful surgeries), a surgeon may have poor customer ratings. While online ratings are useful for gauging some aspects of the patient experience, such as the service-related aspects, they are plainly insufficient for determining if the care provided is of good quality.

It appears that online evaluations have too much influence on how patients make decisions. The fact that a doctor has received high ratings does not suggest that his or her patients have a greater chance of survival.

The scores may not accurately reflect whether a doctor is "excellent" in the medical area. Doctors may be ranked based on whether or not they were able to provide what the patients wanted, rather than on doing what is best for their health, which is one of the greatest review warning flags.

Consider the following example: Researchers at UC Davis Health monitored over 1,700 requests made by patients to their doctors in a recent study. When their wishes were met, which happened around 85 percent of the time, patients were generally satisfied with clinicians.

Patients' satisfaction with their physicians dropped by 10 to 20 percentile points when their requests for referrals, prescriptions, and testing were rejected. This shows that doctors may feel compelled to give antibiotics even if they are reasonably convinced that the pills are not necessary.

The Internet is awash with online ratings, and it is nearly impossible to ignore them. It is understandable that people facing the tough choice of undergoing surgery would want to learn more about their surgeon. Until recently, the majority of physician ratings were based on patient feedback and personal experiences. The Internet is the most common and untrustworthy source of information now.

Let us face it, likes and testimonies can both be purchased. The newer Internet behemoths demand payment from doctors to promote their names alongside the products. Newer physicians have little option but to surrender to this practice, which results in them paying nearly a third of their consultation fee to online aggregators in exchange for patient flow directed toward them.

Although the Internet provides a fair playing field for all doctors to some extent, it is significantly slanted in favour of doctors who pay more promotion fees.

Many people rely on websites that allow patients to rate and review doctors to help them pick a doctor or evaluate their present one, but the information on these sites can be deceptive. Many physician-rating websites (PRWs) include erroneous information giving rise to data quality concerns. According to studies, 53 percent of the sites had intrinsic data quality flaws (accuracy, objectivity, repute, and credibility), whereas 61 percent had contextual data quality difficulties (relevance, value addition, timeliness, and completeness). There were also other issues, such as difficult-to-understand system interfaces and questions about data security and safety.

The following were the most prevalent issues: (a) A striking lack of negative evaluations or comments that are emotionally heated—ratings given anonymously that were not totally credible.

(b) Physicians who paid a premium were able to conceal up to three bad remarks, as well as a low number of reviews and ratings. (c) Positive evaluations based on variables other than physician attributes (ease of getting an appointment, short wait time, or staff behaviors).

(d) Higher ratings were linked to marketing efforts: the placement of good reviews and rating data on the first pages had an influence on patient perception. (e) The use of many scales to assess physicians made the data difficult to comprehend.

Consumer decision-making is heavily influenced by e-WOM, and healthcare is no exception. According to reports, 35 percent of patients chose doctors based on positive reviews, while 37 percent avoided doctors with negative reviews. There are, however, a variety of price rates available.

Working sites occasionally offer doctors the option of purchasing a premium subscription, which gives them more control over the data and reviews that are released. With the purchase of a premium subscription, several sites provided physicians the chance to erase a few unfavorable comments or post advertisements that can affect their ranking in search results. As a result, patients' perceptions are influenced, and their healthcare decisions are influenced.

Make sure you cross-reference the material on different PRWs (Physician rating websites) and verify the physician's background information before making a judgment about a doctor based on an online review.

Although PRWs have certain positive traits, they also have several flaws. Many patients, in particular, may read physician ratings and reviews, but few take the time to post one. According to the study, 37 percent of Internet users have reviewed items and services online, while just 3 percent to 4 percent have reviewed a doctor or a hospital. Because of the low percentage of involvement, there are fewer ratings/reviews per physician, resulting in reports that are less representative of the medical spectrum and more erratic.

The effects of a single negative assessment on the total score can lower the average score and make a high-performing physician seem ordinary.

PRWs do not check the legitimacy of the ratings because of patient privacy concerns; in many cases, a valid e-mail address is the sole condition for rating a physician. In the absence of the ability to verify if ratings/reviews are genuinely supplied by valid patients, there is an obvious risk of harm or fraud, which is frequently perpetrated by patients with a grudge or by those who operate competitive services. Positive reviews, on the other hand, may be written by office employees or particular physicians in order to improve their online reputation. Another point of contention is the veracity of Internet reviews.

Some physicians are incorrectly categorized, while others may have relocated, and their new information has not been updated on the PRWs. Physicians are also worried that circumstances beyond their control may have an impact on their composite score. The patient population serviced appears to have an impact on response rates and ratings. There is evidence that physicians who care for patients from poorer socioeconomic origins may be ranked lower. These concerns raise the possibility that physicians would be improperly rewarded or penalized for treating certain patient groups, resulting in a decline in care for vulnerable patients.

Patients are also referred to surgeons by their general practitioners or family physicians. These physicians would usually have a long association with the patients' families and feel obligated to them. Patients in the United Kingdom may not have a choice and may be referred to a hospital, where they will be visited by any surgeon who is available at the time, and he may or may not be the one who operates on them eventually.

In nations like India, however, primary care doctors have a choice and are frequently accused of accepting bribes from hospitals and surgeons. Because of these arrangements, this style of reference is frequently untrustworthy.

However, it may be one of the input techniques to some extent since family physicians do not want patients returning with issues and blaming them for deceiving them. Doctors throughout India are united in their belief that "kickbacks and bribes that grease every element of the healthcare system" are a major factor.

In many five-star corporate hospitals, where the main motive appears to be not just patient care, doctors have been confronted by the hospital management asking them to justify the salary they were drawing. Not all hospitals do that, and having worked in Apollo hospitals for 20 years now, never have I been confronted by a member of the management regarding the salary that I draw. Many believe that the widespread practice of bribery is linked to the private health sector, which has grown to dominate healthcare in India and is now clamouring for a market share. They also believe that doctors should be given a full-time wage under a nationalized healthcare program, such as exists in the United Kingdom, so that there is no motivation for them to propose unnecessary operations or investigations.

The corruption in healthcare industry, inevitably result from intense competition, intense investment, and intense saturation. It is much more than just a moral or ethical concern. It is a free-for-all approach to medicine, with unrestrained expansion and significant investment. If there are five CT scan centers within a one-kilometer radius, they are competing for the same market.

Such activity is tightly restricted in several nations. Reversing such a high level of privatization would need political will, but we may use rigorous deterrence to put an end to such behaviours. It needs to come from within the industry. The fact that such wrongdoings are difficult to establish is one of the main reasons for their increasing bravado. In this practice, there is no definite data.

However, the bulk of referrals is based on fee-splitting. This goes against the grain of practicing medicine, which exists to serve a societal purpose in the form of healthcare. The medical profession's reputation and legitimacy are slowly eroding.

Having said that there is a corrupt system within the healthcare industry, it must also be mentioned that there are a number of hospitals and surgeons who follow a proper and ethical medical practice where patient care is the top agenda. How else can we explain the tremendous increase in medical tourism seen in India in the last decade alone!

Healthcare has become expensive and the government has not been able to come to the rescue of the common man. It became amply clear in the ongoing pandemic where the private hospitals had to be arm twisted to give up almost 80 percent of their hospital beds for government-referred patients. At present, the government spends just 1 percent of the GDP on healthcare, whereas we need to spend at least 6 percent if we are to come within sight of what the National Health Service (NHS, the UK healthcare system) is doing. A Da Vinci robotic system costs about 22 crores, which includes training for the surgeons. How will a hospital recover the cost of the surgery? They have to charge the patient or the insurance company. Going by the numbers, a robotic prostate surgery would cost about 4000 USD in India. Whereas in the USA, it would easily cost 11,000 USD to 25,000 USD (in 2016). People are looking for world-class healthcare at Indian costs! How is it possible? Going by the cost breakup, the surgeon would get a mere 11 percent to 13 percent of the total bill in a corporate hospital. The simple fact is that we lost the plot the day we started referring to the healthcare system as a health care industry and the patient became a consumer!

That is where the fault line lies! You cannot call it 'industry' and then not go by the free growth and support standards, which are enjoyed by the other sectors, such as the IT sector.

However, it is true that the instances of bribery and corruption are not static. Perhaps there are physicians who have been treating you since antiquity or who have their IKIGAI sorted, and their only concern is your health. They will definitely be suggesting to you the surgeons who are best qualified to fix your health condition. The ratings are not always the options by which you can select your surgeons. If you are not sure what sort of surgeon you require, contact your physician or a specialist. Some procedures, such as appendectomy, may be performed by a general surgeon, while others require the expertise of a specialist.

Due to the lucrative nature of plastic surgery and cosmetic operations, there have been several incidents of fraud involving people posing as plastic surgeons, including genuine physicians who have never been trained in plastic surgery but perform aesthetic procedures. You really do not have to go very far for this practice. Just switch on your television and see how many small centers are offering procedures like hair transplants, adding to the patients' confusion.

If you feel comfortable discussing your surgery preparations with others and you know someone who has had a comparable procedure, inquire about their surgeon. Would they recommend their surgeon to a friend? Your acquaintance will be able to tell you whether they were properly prepared for the procedure and provided with all of the information they needed to make an educated decision. Do not forget to ask about their experience with the surgical facility as well. If you need highly specialized surgery, do not be surprised if the surgeon recommended is in a different part of the state.

Unless you reside in a major city, you may not be able to obtain treatment close to home if the surgical procedure you need is a rare one. Just keep in mind that the ultimate result is more important than your surgeon's bedside manner.

Choose the skillful surgeon over the charming surgeon if you have to choose between the two. Hopefully, you will succeed in finding someone who is kind as well as competent. If you reside in a small town, the number of surgeons available to you may be restricted.

If your alternatives are too restricted, get a list for the next big city and see if the number of surgeons available expands. Compare the names suggested by your family doctor, friends, relatives, and other sources to the names on the insurance company's list. Make a note if the names of any of the surgeons who were suggested appear on your insurance list.

Even if you are having an elective treatment that your insurance will not cover, such as cosmetic surgery, you should still get your insurance company's list since it will help you create a list of doctors to choose from. In a nutshell, you want a surgeon who has performed the treatment so many times that they are highly comfortable with it and whose team is confident in their abilities to care for patients before, during, and after the process.

Now the question is how will you decide who is the best surgeon to treat your health condition.

After much deliberation, and examining hundreds of inputs in form of questioners and survey-monkey forms from patients, we have developed a algorithm to help you make an informed decision. Especially when you have time before your surgical procedure. You could use this algorithm to reach the correct person for your or your relative's surgery. It looks at various aspect and sources of information that a patient may receive in order to make an informed decision and then gives them creditably points according to their importance. WOM gets the highest creditability and importance as that source is the gold standard. Others too get points according to their creditability and trueness of the data that they provide. The final score will give you an answer: How to choose your surgeon! Happy hunting!

| Values | Credits | Surgeon A | Surgeon B | Surgeon C | Surgeon D | Surgeon E |
|---|---|---|---|---|---|---|
| Education | 1-4 | | | | | |
| Experience | 1-3 | | | | | |
| Availability | 1-3 | | | | | |
| Behavior | 1-3 | | | | | |
| Personality | 1-2 | | | | | |
| Word of mouth | 1-4 | | | | | |
| Internet likes | 1-2 | | | | | |
| Ikigai | 1-3 | | | | | |
| Written Testimonials | 1-2 | | | | | |
| Video Testimonials | 1-4 | | | | | |
| Total | | | | | | |

# 6

# FROM BURP TO FART, WE HAVE IT COVERED

## General And Gastrointestinal Surgery

*"The only weapon with which the unconscious patient can immediately retaliate upon the incompetent surgeon is hemorrhage."*
– William Stewart Halsted

India is a vast country with great diversity. There are differences in the languages, diets, and sleeping patterns of its population. This diversity is not just in terms of how it differs from other countries, but also within itself. However, one of the best examples of how it differs from the rest of the world is in its medical facilities. The training that potential surgeons undergo in India varies across regions.

If you were to look at countries like the US and the UK, medical training is protocol-based. It is not the case in India. If you were to look at some of the premier institutions like the Indian Institute of Medical Sciences or JIPMER, Puducherry, the training will be extensive and exhaustive.

Veer away from these central institutes and go to some of the less fancied medical colleges, and you will find that the training is far from adequate. Medical training in India is not uniform across its medical colleges.

Hence, when India produces a new batch of doctors and surgeons, they come with a varied set of skills and experiences. The relevant question here is this: Does it matter if they graduate as differently-trained doctors? Perhaps a quote by Moshe Schein would give you the answer: The most important clotting factor is the surgeon.

The skills honed by a surgeon are based on their training and experience. If the skills vary, there will be a natural difference in clinical outcomes. The greatest difference in training comes in the field of general surgery and its related branches. Why? It is best understood by breaking it down into numbers. There are about 1200 seats for general surgery in India. There are 1499 super specialization seats (MCh) in India. There are the same number of Diplomate in National Board (DNB) seats too. DNB is a post-graduate degree equivalent to that of a Master's degree. Doctorate of National Board (DrNB) is a super specialty degree equivalent to a DM or MCh degree. Doctors undergo DNB and DrNB training in their chosen specialty or super specialty, usually in private hospitals, such as Sir Ganga Ram Hospital.

Those who obtain an MCh or DrNB degree go on to become specialists in neurosurgery, urology, cardiothoracic surgery, etc. On completion of their Master's in general surgery, surgeons would know their Ikigai by then and decide the branch of specialization they wish to pursue. Most of the surgeons opt for gastrointestinal (GI) surgery, urology, onco-surgery, or neurosurgery. Other branches like cardiothoracic and vascular surgery, plastic surgery, and pediatric surgery have seats lying vacant even in premier institutions, such as Jayadeva Institute of Cardiology in Bangalore, for want of takers! There are multiple issues why certain seats are more attractive than others. We will look into those reasons at a later stage.

One of the biggest challenges in India is to determine how well-trained a surgeon is. Where did a particular surgeon study? Does the said surgeon's medical college train its students appropriately? Was there adequate mentorship? It is difficult for recruiters to determine the capacity of a surgeon.

There could be an obvious bias like believing that a surgeon from a lesser-known institution would have undergone a lower standard of training, which may not always be true. However, what if the said surgeon worked harder than someone from an elite college to make up for the difference?

Just imagine the difficulty for patients when recruiters themselves struggle to make a decision about surgeons. They just cannot determine the quality and potential of a surgeon.

So, the recruiters do not look at the college of a potential hire. What they could look at instead are the raw numbers.

What was the caseload for the surgeon? How many patients died at his hands? How many operations did they participate in? How many surgeries did the surgeon independently perform?

It is important here to clarify the training of a surgeon. All the surgical super-specialists have to first undergo the MBBS (Bachelor of Medicine and Bachelor of Surgery) training. This is followed by an MS (Master of Surgery) in general surgery. It is when they graduate from the latter course that they become eligible to appear in the entrance exam and join the elite group of super-specialist doctors and surgeons like urologists, cardiothoracic surgeons, pediatric surgeons, onco-surgeons, etc.

A general surgeon, on graduating from the MS course, is generally considered to be 'under-cooked' in surgical expertise. Hence, it is always a good idea for the newly qualified general surgeon to join a competent team under the mentorship of a senior surgeon for further training. It is much like pilot training. Having a license does not mean the pilot can fly a Boeing 777 from day one! They can learn from senior surgeons and build up a caseload and have varied experiences. Once they build up enough experience, they can start their independent consultancy.

However, this is not the case in India, especially in private hospitals. Many surgeons begin immediately as they would have a father, mother, or relative to ease them into such jobs. It is extremely difficult to find out how many surgeries were performed by a surgeon and, of course, there is no prescribed method to investigate and find out.

The primary reason for the lack of information is the absence of a database that lists the surgeries performed during training and afterward. Although there is an effort now for the surgeons to maintain a logbook, the books can be cooked and there is no way of knowing how many 'real' hands-on surgeries a surgeon has performed before passing out. Many medical colleges in India have very few patients. There are not enough cases for a student to be trained. This is the irony of the system, which has a huge population and empty hospitals.

Most of the patients choose to spend out of their pocket, selling their lands and houses, to pay for treatment at private hospitals, simply because they do not trust the government medical system. At this point, it becomes a pressing question for patients. Where will they go? There is such a vast difference in the training a surgeon receives.

How does a patient choose from among an ill-trained surgeon, a slightly-trained surgeon, a well-trained surgeon, and an extremely well-trained surgeon?

The extremely well-trained surgeon, without doubt, will have the best clinical outcome. But how can a patient identify and differentiate between these surgeons? The general rule seems to be based on the degree (MS or MCh) of the surgeon. People look at their qualifications (specialisation and super specialisation) and assign value to the qualification that the surgeon possesses. Most patients use this criterion as a thumb rule to select a surgeon. Surgery is a skill and this criterion may be totally misleading as the best-qualified surgeon may have a poor skill set. At this point, let me explain more clearly the journey of a surgeon. There are two types of surgeons with super specialisation practicing in India.

The first group has those who obtained their qualifications in India and the other group has those who obtained their super specialisation degree abroad. If I were just a general surgeon, I would not be able to make enough money to make ends meet. I would be performing some surgical procedures, but they would not pay as well as the super-specialty surgeries would. An average Indian patient looks for more than a general surgeon. So, most Indian surgeons look to do a specialisation as well to give them an edge over the others.

I specialised in one of the most esteemed medical institutions in medical history. It was the Mayo Clinic in Rochester, USA. I specialised in Bariatric surgery. The Mayo Clinic was ranked the second-best medical institution in the world. My eyes were opened due to the number of cases I was exposed to at Mayo. I had an excellent mentor in Dr. Jeff Thompson.

He was extremely kind and generous with his time and trained me extremely well. When I passed out of the institute, I was a changed man. If you were to look at it technically, my skills had not undergone any great transformation. The transformational change came about in my perspective. My mental horizons had expanded. I had become a Bariatric Surgeon.

Bariatric surgery is a form of laparoscopic surgery or GI surgery. It is done on extremely obese patients. It is very challenging to conduct a keyhole surgery in such patients. However, as I built up my expertise in bariatric surgery, I realized something very important.

As I kept performing these extremely difficult surgeries under trying circumstances, the other abdominal surgeries became easier to perform.

When I came upon this realisation, my horizons expanded. I knew that I could go beyond being a general surgeon or a laparoscopic surgeon.

There was a sea change in my vision. My transformation from a general surgeon to a laparoscopic surgeon, and then finally to a bariatric surgeon, and later to a robotic surgeon was very challenging.

As per the NLM Medical Subject Headings, laparoscopy is defined as, "A procedure in which a laparoscope (laparoscopes) is inserted through a small incision near the navel to examine the abdominal and pelvic organs in the peritoneal cavity. If appropriate, biopsy or surgery can be performed during laparoscopy. Essentially, it is a surgery performed with minimum incisions—minimally invasive surgery or laparoscopic surgery. I completed my MS in a government medical college at Udaipur. There were many open surgery cases. Keyhole surgeries were rare but the surgical training was robust. I was always attracted to laparoscopic surgery and so I decided to go to the place where most of the action was happening in the laparoscopy space. Finally, I got the chance to become a registrar at Sir Ganga Ram Hospital (SGRH).

Six months prior to joining SGRH, I had never dreamt of the possibility of even holding a laparoscope in my hands, much less performing laparoscopic surgery on my own. However, I was blessed with the best and kindest professors and bosses, and awesome colleagues.

Perhaps they saw and recognised my passion and my potential or maybe this was just how they were! They gave me enough opportunities to perform independent laparoscopic surgeries to build up sufficient confidence in me to go out and start my own practice. I managed to do it despite finding Delhi to be an overwhelming place. It was not easy as this was the time when I was also starting a family. (In India we do everything together: getting married, having children, getting trained with 36 hours on-call duties, and also trying to get a life!) Not a good match at all. But then when my peers could do it, why can't I? Again, a wrong analogy to base my life on. If I had to live my life again, I would do things a bit differently. I started my independent practice in Jaipur. To my surprise, there were not many surgeons who were trained in laparoscopy.

I built up my expertise with many more successful cases and a good reputation, and with a little luck, the opportunity of lifetime came knocking. I got the chance to go to the Mayo Clinic.

When I returned from Mayo Clinic, I got the opportunity to start my practice at Apollo Hospital in Goa. I had trained myself in laparoscopic surgery and bariatric surgery.

I was a different surgeon from the one who had started out five years ago from a government hospital in Udaipur. I no longer baulked at the idea of doing laparoscopic hemicolectomies, keyhole surgeries for the stomach, liver, and pancreas, or splenic surgeries. I no longer found them difficult. The reason was my expertise in bariatric surgery. It is considered the benchmark when it comes to challenging laparoscopic surgeries.

*"Every surgeon carries within himself a small cemetery, where from time to time he goes to pray..."* – Rene Leriche

The Rene Leriche quote may seem dark, but it is indicative of the growth of a surgeon. My journey from being a general surgeon to a bariatric surgeon was never easy. It was a painful journey. There is the pain of learning, the pain of delivering results, the pain of getting your own patient base, and the pain of building a meaningful relationship of trust with your patients. Then there is the pain of constant learning and upgrading your knowledge and skills. This journey is not unique to me alone. Every surgeon has to traverse this path. And like every surgeon, I would not have it any other way. I grew and evolved through these experiences. The words of Richard Selzer epitomize my feeling exactly: "And if the surgeon is like a poet, then the scars you have made on countless bodies are like verses into the fashioning of which you have poured your soul."

However, there are many instances where a surgeon can be overwhelmed with the amount of learning. There will be surgeons who wish to stop the lengthy learning process and start their own practice. My learning curve was also long. I was 37 years old when I finished learning bariatric surgery at the Mayo Clinic.

If you were to look at a software engineer comparatively, they would be at the top of their career at the age of 37. Here, at the age of 37, I was at the starting line.

I also got an opportunity at that time to be a consultant at Apollo Hospital in Bangalore. I was now considered trained well enough to deliver good clinical outcomes consistently.

I started my medical career as an MBBS student at the age of 18. It took me the same amount of time to be considered trustworthy enough to deliver as a bariatric surgeon. I had spent more than half of my life to reach this point. It was tedious and I felt every moment of those 18-odd years. Every surgeon I know has had to go through this journey. There are a few surgeons who do not like to go through this long journey. They would like to go to more specialised centres like JIPMER for training in GI surgery and get an MCh (Magister Chirurgiae) in GI surgery. It is considered one of the premier degrees to be obtained in India and guarantees placement and patient following.

Comparatively speaking, those who would opt for the MCh degree would find it easier than my journey. They are definitely the brightest of the lot and it is really difficult to get into one of these programmmes, and once in the system, the training is hard and grueling. They are trained to undertake the most difficult abdominal surgeries, such as liver transplantation and pancreatic malignancy surgeries. Surgeons with an MCh have it easier as the degree on its own guarantees them sufficient patient load of many easier surgeries. A surgeon with an MCh degree is associated with the idea of reliability and the promise of delivering by default due to the brand value of the degree.

However, that is not the case for surgeons like me. I have to deliver and provide evidence of my skill. I have to prove myself. This conflict is experienced by all the surgeons who have trod my path. It is true for those who went before me and for those who will come after me as well. However, the fault does not lie with the surgeons. The fault lies with the system in India. If you were to look at the Western countries, their system is completely different.

After our Western counterparts complete their MS, their super specialisation is organ specific.

So, you will find surgeons who carry different designations and specialisations. They are Upper GI Surgeons, Colorectal Surgeons, Hepatobiliary Surgeons, or Bariatric Surgeons. These specialisations follow their basic training and, as mentioned earlier, are organ-specific. The Western system is better organised and allows surgeons to narrow their focus on one type of surgery and become better by repetition. In contrast, if you were to be a GI surgeon with an MCh degree, you would become a jack-of-all-trades and master of none unless you decide to focus your energies on only one organ. Although the referral system in India is not robust enough to feed one type of surgery to a surgeon, it appears to be the best alternative, and a sound referral system is the need of the hour.

The Indian system with such wide definitions of surgeons is bound to fail in the future. This statement might seem like an exaggeration. However, this is the reality of the situation. As mentioned earlier, there is a lot more nuance and detail involved when it comes to being an organ-specific surgeon. This system can befuddle patients into the perception that GI surgeons are just better trained general surgeons. However, this system is equally harmful to the surgeons as well. A surgeon with an MCh in GI surgery would be in direct competition with a trained surgeon like myself and there lies the bias in the system!

Then there are other conflicts at play as well. A patient, quite understandably, will want a well-established surgeon as that designation will suggest the highest guarantee of delivering success. Let us imagine this scenario. Let us say a patient has been operated upon by a general surgeon with specialised training, quite similar to my case. The operation is a success. However, if the same patient is then offered a GI surgeon with an MCh degree for another abdomen operation, who will he choose? I have no answer to that question as I am not sure of the patient's choice. This is the kind of confusion that this system has caused. These topics have fueled many intense discussions between me and my colleagues.

We have tried to rationalise our patient in-flows and have failed.

Surgeons who underwent experiences similar to mine would attest to the importance of narrowing our focus. But this is the nature of the flawed system in India. It is chaotic and ridden with conflicts.

It is within such a system that a patient has to choose a surgeon. A patient can be faced with quite a dilemma when it comes to choosing a surgeon. He could either choose a general surgeon with specialised training in laparoscopic surgery or other organ-specific surgery or a general surgeon who has an MCh degree in GI surgery. To stir the pot further, there could be foreign-trained surgeons either from the UK (FRCS) or from the US (MD) who have specialised and trained in particular surgeries like colorectal surgeries and hepatobiliary surgeries. Although well trained, these surgeons face a lot of difficulty in India, when they try to set up an independent practice here as there is no specific referral system in India. The Indian system also does not recognise their degrees except for the private hospitals.

This is the problem of choice that an Indian patient faces in this country. So, how does a patient choose a surgeon in India? The thumb rule is by looking at the degrees or relying on word of mouth.

They also look at the position held by the surgeon in the hospital. They will trust a well-established senior surgeon from a large hospital. However, objectively speaking, this may not be the best choice for the patient. There may be many junior surgeons who fill in the consultant roles at large hospitals who are doing a sufficiently acceptable job. The clinical outcomes may not be uniform in such a mix. These surgeons could be a little cavalier in their outlook and may still be in the 'testing my boundaries' stage.

I find this quote by Stanley O Hoerr particularly relevant here: *"The surgeon is a man of action. By temperament and by training he prefers to serve the sick by operating on them, and he inwardly commiserates with a patient so unfortunate as to have a disease not suited to surgical treatment. Young surgeons, busy mastering the technicalities of the art, are particularly alert to seize every legitimate opportunity to practice technical maneuvers, the more complicated the better."*

These surgeons will push themselves and could end up having complications. This would then cause them to go into their shells and then they could stop taking chances. The consequence is that they would not gather enough experience. The system will tell them not to take chances as complications mean loss of revenue. This is how the Indian private healthcare system functions. Of course, there are hospitals like SGRH that may provide them with a longer rope as complications may not necessarily point to a lack of skill or experience in a surgeon.

It could also point to problems in the infrastructure or the environment would not have been conducive for the complex surgery. I am reminded of a liver transplant operation that happened in the early 2000s at a reputed hospital in New Delhi. It was the first one of its kind and I happened to witness the operation. Unfortunately, the patient did not make it.

When it comes to such complicated surgeries, there could be a number of factors at play. The hospital machinery may not have been well oiled, the postoperative care may not have been adequate as no one had the experience in dealing with such patients, or the patient's body may have rejected the transplant. It could be any one of these factors or a combination of all. It does not always boil down to the surgeon's skill or experience. A surgeon can only do so much. I am not sure how this surgeon would have fared if he were in any other private medical institution. Would he have been asked to stop participating in other complicated surgeries?

This hospital gave him the opportunity to grow and improve with experience. Today, he is an extremely reputed transplant surgeon in Delhi. This is how the GI surgeons differ from one another. They could have taken the route of going to a reputed medical institution and getting trained for an MCh degree. They could have also taken an alternate but longer route to specialise in specific-organ surgeries. Even though I took the latter route, I will not claim that one surgeon is superior to the other. So, if you are a patient, you will have a pertinent question: "How do I choose the right surgeon for my GI problem?"

There is a common misconception that there is no place for humour or lightheartedness in our profession as general surgeons and GI surgeons. Nothing could be further from the truth. Well, it is true that there are unwritten rules about how surgeons should behave with their patients in operation theatres and OPDs. It is not considered the 'done thing' to show our emotions openly when dealing with patients, and etiquette demands that we keep our emotions under control.

But despite our best efforts, we do sometimes crack a smile at some of the patients who come to see us. I remember a patient who was referred to me by my friend, a neurosurgeon. The patient came to my OPD with a strange complaint. He was sure there was a microchip in his mind or body, and he was unable to locate it. He felt he was being controlled by this chip from head to toe. Apparently, the chip had been implanted by an alien while he was asleep.

Now, my friend, the neurosurgeon, has a mischievous side to him and decided he would let me deal with this problem. He sent a referral note stating he had ruled out the presence of any chip in the mind, and it was probably in the GI tract. He conveyed this to the patient and sent him to my OPD.

When I heard the patient's account, my first thought was to send him for a psychiatric evaluation. Obviously, this was an ailment not to be found in any medical or surgical textbook. I tried hard to keep a straight face as I told this patient that it was possible and that it would take extensive investigations to locate it. An MRI might be needed, and possibly even that might fail to pick it up. I was trying to be empathetic and slowly lead the conversation to the possibility of a psychiatric evaluation.

It was all I could do to hold back my smile. This was the first instance when someone had been referred to me for the removal of an imaginary chip from their abdomen.

There was another instance in my career when I totally lost control and laughed at what the patient was telling me. A gentleman came to my OPD and said he had a problem with his 'bowling.'

Being a GI surgeon, I wondered why this patient came to me if he had a problem in his arm while bowling in a game of cricket. So, I asked who had sent him to me. He answered, "I thought you looked after the bowling problems." I was puzzled, and then it struck me—he was talking about 'bowel movements.' It had nothing to do with cricket and everything to do with constipation!

Just as the light dawned, the patient made a gesture to show the kind of 'bowling' he was referring to. That did it—I burst out laughing! That was the first and the last time that I actually laughed in front of a patient. Needless to say, that patient went away and never came back to me.

Over the years, we have schooled ourselves not to show our emotions. Whatever ridiculous question or explanation is put to us by a patient, we keep a straight face and answer them.

"The world runs on feelings" as the author of the book Everything Is F*cked: A Book About Hope, Mark Manson, puts it. Ultimately the vibe that you get from a particular surgeon will decide if you want him to work on you! For other people who want their rational brain to do the job, we have devised an algorithm to help you make that choice.

Score your choices based on the chapters you have read so far on the table below. Go with the surgeon who scores the highest.

| Values | Credits | Surgeon A | Surgeon B | Surgeon C | Surgeon D | Surgeon E |
|---|---|---|---|---|---|---|
| Education | 1-4 | | | | | |
| Experience | 1-3 | | | | | |
| Availability | 1-3 | | | | | |
| Behaviour | 1-3 | | | | | |
| Personality | 1-2 | | | | | |
| Word of mouth | 1-4 | | | | | |
| Internet likes | 1-2 | | | | | |
| Ikigai | 1-3 | | | | | |
| Testimonials | 1-2 | | | | | |
| Video-Testimonials | 1-4 | | | | | |
| Total | | | | | | |

# 7
# ROUND IS ALSO A SHAPE
## Bariatric Surgery

Not a Magic Cure.

Most people would be familiar with the term 'Bariatric Surgery.' It is more commonly known as weight-loss surgery. Being a Bariatric surgeon, this subject is close to my heart and is dealt with a little more elaborately. There is an interesting anecdote quoted in Spanish history.[1] The first bariatric procedure was apparently performed in the 10th century CE in Spain and the first patient to undergo the procedure is said to have been the King of Leon, Sancho. Apparently, he was so obese that he was unable to even walk. Obviously, it follows that he could neither ride a horse nor take part in a swordfight, which led to him losing his throne. His grandmother is said to have taken him to the famous Jewish doctor, Hasdai Ibn Shaprut, in Cordoba. The good doctor sutured the king's lips together such that there was just a small gap for a straw to be inserted.

The king was thus fed mainly a liquid diet with a few herbs to stimulate weight loss. King Sancho is said to have lost half his weight and to have returned on horseback to Leon to reclaim his throne successfully. If only it were so simple! So let us look at what exactly is bariatric surgery and how it helps in weight loss. **Bariatric surgery versus Cosmetic surgery** Bariatric surgery refers to certain surgical procedures that are performed on the gastrointestinal (GI) tract in people who are overweight. In simple terms, these surgical procedures result in decreased absorption of calories from the GI tract and an early feeling of satiety. People often confuse bariatric surgery with cosmetic surgery.[2] Cosmetic surgery is where certain procedures are performed to remove existing fat cells to make the patient look better. The various cosmetic surgical procedures include removal of abdominal fat, liposuction, tummy tucks, and body contouring. These cosmetic measures only serve to improve body shape and enhance the physical appearance of people. They give a psychological boost to people who have increased fat deposits in specific areas of their bodies. Cosmetic procedures in no way address the main cause of obesity in the patient, and they do not have any role in aiding the patient to maintain weight loss over a period of time. The actual amount of weight loss achieved through cosmetic procedures is minuscule compared to that achieved with a bariatric surgical procedure. It is said that a cosmetic surgery procedure can help in an average weight loss of less than 2 kg to 10 kg. Bariatric surgery, on the other hand, addresses the root cause of obesity. Factors that lead to obesity in a particular patient are identified and the issue of long-term weight loss is tackled. Patients undergoing bariatric surgery can look to a weight loss of around 55 kg to 70 kg or sometimes even up to 200 kg. Bariatric surgical measures also help in managing various co-morbidities that may be present in an obese individual, such as diabetes and hypertension as well as other obesity-related health issues.

In short, cosmetic surgery does not have any impact on thegeneral health of the patient. whereas bariatric surgery aids in addressing multiple health issues associated with obesity in patients.

## Obesity and its Attendant Woes

What is obesity and why is it important? Obesity is basically a condition where there is excess fat in the body leading to an increase in the weight of the person. The measure of obesity is the body mass index (BMI). The BMI is based on the height and weight of the person and applies to adults. It is calculated using the formula $BMI=kg/m2$, where kg stands for a person's weight in kilograms and m2 stands for their height in meters squared. The BMI is used to grade obesity. In adults who are 20 years of age or older, a BMI of below 18.5 indicates underweight status, 18.5 to 24.9 indicates a healthy weight, 25.0 to 29.9 indicates that the person is overweight, and 30.0 and above indicates obesity. Obesity, in turn, is graded as obese, severely obese, and morbidly obese. The health risks to the person also increase with an increase in the BMI above the normal values.

### Causes of obesity:
Overeating
Sedentary lifestyle and lack of physical activity
Genetic susceptibility
Endocrine causes
Certain medications
Many more causes are yet to be identified. In fact, there are 60 varieties of obesity and so many influencing factors. It is important to address the issue of obesity, especially in patients who are severely or morbidly obese, because it can result in a lot of health issues.
### Consequences of obesity:
Type 2 diabetes
Hypertension
Heart disease

Gall bladder disease

Certain cancers

Breathing problems.

Fertility issues

Urinary incontinence

Arthritis of the joints

Shorter life expectancy.

There are new issues related to obesity being identified every day, such as COVID patients who were obese had a 20 percent higher mortality when compared to that of patients with normal weight. Obese patients may also experience psychological issues, such as negative body image, social discrimination, and depression.

They may experience difficulties in carrying out activities of daily living, keeping up with their professional life, maintaining personal hygiene, and moving from place to place.

Owing to all these health consequences, it is important to address the issue of obesity effectively. There are many ways to do this, and always the non-surgical conservative measures are tried first. These include dieting, exercise regimes, hormone replacement if required, lifestyle modifications, and such. However, in certain patients who are severely or morbidly obese, none of these measures work and a surgical solution seems to be the only option, that is, bariatric surgery.

## Bariatric Surgical Procedures

The first instance of a bariatric or metabolic surgery in modern medical practice was reported to have been performed by Kremen in 1954 (1). He performed a jejuno-ileal bypass procedure where he simply took one part of the intestine and attached it to another, a little further away, causing food not to traverse the intestine.

This food is bypassed and does not contribute to the absorption of any foodstuff. In 1966, Dr. Mason, a surgeon from the University of Iowa, proposed gastric bypass surgery as the first bariatric surgery.

Since then, several modifications and improvements have been made to the original procedure and newer methods have come into practice as well. These procedures are presently performed using small incisions and minimally invasive surgical techniques, such as laparoscopy or robotics.

Basically, these procedures help a person achieve a healthy body weight by decreasing the absorption of nutrients or decreasing hunger, and promoting early satiety.

In general, bariatric surgery either reduces the size of the stomach so that after surgery the person feels like they have eaten enough quickly, or a malabsorptive condition is created where only a portion of the food that is eaten is digested and turned into calories, or a combination of both.

The commonly performed bariatric surgical procedures that are recognized by the Obesity and Metabolic Surgery Society of India (OSSI) are the following[34]

Gastric Bypass Surgery or the Roux-en-Y procedure: This surgical procedure is considered the oldest among all bariatric surgeries. This procedure can be performed laparoscopically under general anesthesia. The laparoscope with camera and light attachments is inserted through an incision on the abdominal wall. The surgeon views the internal organs on a monitor.

Surgical instruments are inserted through other incisions made on the abdominal wall. In this procedure, the stomach is stapled and a small pouch is created at the superior aspect.

This pouch is then directly anastomosed to the lower section of the small intestine, creating a 'roux limb.' The digestive juices from the remaining portion of the stomach drain into the upper section of the small intestine, which is attached to the distal end of the 'roux limb.' This basically results in food bypassing the stomach and directly entering the small intestine.

This can be termed as a combined procedure, that is, the amount of food eaten will be less and also absorption of nutrients will be impaired. This in turn decreases hunger, increases fullness, and helps the body to attain the ideal weight. This bariatric surgical procedure is also said to improve type 2 diabetes in patients.

Advantages: (a) The weight loss is long-lasting. (b) It helps in the management of other obesity-related health conditions. (c) The technique has been in practice for many years and is standardized. (d) Surgeons have gained experience in performing this technique over many decades.

Disadvantages: (a) It is a slightly more complex surgical procedure compared to the other two procedures. (b) The patient may experience more vitamin and mineral deficiencies. (c) There is a post-surgical risk of small bowel obstruction and other complications. (d) Patients who undergo this procedure should be careful about tobacco use or the ingestion of non-steroidal anti-inflammatory drugs. (e) Patients may experience the 'Dumping Syndrome.'

This involves a feeling of indigestion and sickness immediately after eating or drinking something, especially hard-to-digest foods like sweets. (f) Leaks may develop in the GI tract. (g) Patients may develop hernias, gallstones, and ulcers.**Gastric Banding:**

This procedure involves the placing of an inflatable silicone band around the upper part of the stomach. The band is inflated using sterile saline till it constricts the stomach optimally. This helps to create a small upper pouch and a larger lower pouch. When food is ingested, the upper pouch fills up quickly and gives a feeling of satiety or fullness to the patient. This aids the patient to reduce his food intake.

This is an adjustable procedure and the level of the band can be changed depending on the amount of food you want the stomach to hold. The access port connected to the band is placed under the skin of the abdomen. This allows the surgeon to inflate or deflate the band as required. This procedure has largely been given up due to band-related complications.

Advantages: (a) This is a less invasive procedure with a shorter hospital stay. (b) Post-surgery complications are minimal. (c) There is no surgical division of the stomach or intestines. (d) The band can be removed when required. It is a reversible procedure. (e) There is minimal risk for vitamin and mineral deficiencies.

Disadvantages: (a) Band adjustment may require the patient to make multiple hospital visits. (b) Weight loss is slower and to a lesser extent with this procedure. (c) Slippage of the band or erosion of the stomach may occur. (d) Internal bleeding and infections may occur. (e) Dilatation of the esophagus may occur.

## Sleeve Gastrectomy

This is a restrictive bariatric surgical procedure used to treat extremely obese patients with a BMI of 40 or above. It is a laparoscopic procedure. Multiple small incisions are made in the abdomen under general anesthesia. The laparoscope with a camera and light attached is inserted through one of the incisions. The surgical instruments are passed through the other incisions. The surgeon views the internal organs on a monitor. In this procedure, a major portion of the stomach (75%–80%) is removed and then the remaining portion is stapled together. All skin incisions are closed with sutures at the end of the procedure. This procedure restricts the amount of food eaten by the patient. The portion of the stomach that produces the hunger hormone is removed, and this affects the metabolism. It decreases the feeling of hunger and increases the feeling of fullness.

Advantages: (a) It is a simpler procedure requiring less time. (b) Normal functions of the stomach are retained. (c) There is minimal postoperative pain and discomfort.

(d) It can be performed in patients who have other high-risk co-morbidities as well.

(e) Patients exhibit significant weight loss and improvement in other obesity-related health conditions as well.

Disadvantages: (a) It is a non-reversible procedure. (b) It can cause postoperative heartburn or acid reflux, for which you may have to take medications. (c) It has a lesser metabolic effect than that seen with gastric bypass procedures.

## Mini Gastric Bypass

This is a short, simple reversible laparoscopic procedure. It is also known as the One Anastomosis Gastric Bypass. This surgery is performed under general anesthesia. The surgeon makes multiple small incisions on the abdomen. The laparoscope is inserted through an incision and the surgeon views the internal organs on a monitor. Instruments are passed through the other incisions to perform the surgery. The size of the stomach is reduced by stapling, leaving a small pouch up to the antrum. Next, a bypass is made for enabling food to move from the new stomach pouch. This is achieved by anastomosing a loop of the small intestine to the newly formed pouch. This loop enables food to bypass the lower portion of the stomach and the duodenum and directly enter the small intestine.

Advantages (a) Short and simple procedure. (b) It involves a shorter hospital stay. (c) It helps resolve obesity-related health conditions. (d) It is a reversible procedure, unlike the Roux-en-Y surgery.

Disadvantages: (a) The area for malabsorption is larger than that seen with regular bypass surgery and this can cause vitamin and mineral deficiencies to a greater extent. (b) Prolonged follow-up care is required to ensure proper diet and nutritional status. (c) Severe complications can occur in certain patients. There are several new and upcoming bariatric surgical procedures being performed worldwide that still need validation from experts around the world. Risks and Complications of Bariatric Surgery -Just like with any surgical procedure, bariatric surgery, too, is associated with its own set of risks and complications.

In general, the more extensive the surgical procedure, the greater the risk of complications occurring.

Patients who have undergone bariatric procedures will require lifelong special monitoring as well as special foods. Complications following bariatric surgery can occur during the procedure, in the immediate postoperative period, or in the long-term postoperative period. Intraoperative complications in bariatric surgical procedures occur rarely and include anesthesia-related events, injury to the abdominal organs, such as bowel, liver, or spleen, and damage to a major blood vessel, such as the inferior vena cava or the portal vein.

Other postoperative complications are listed below:

A small percentage of patients who have undergone weight-loss operations might require follow-up surgery.

Abdominal hernias can occur in these patients, requiring corrective surgery.

Patients may develop gastric leakage through the staples or sutures that were used in the procedure.

Leakage of stomach acids and enzymes can lead to abscess formation and infection in the abdominal cavity.

Patients may develop ulcers in the stomach or small intestine, especially following sleeve gastrectomy procedures. These can lead to chronic abdominal pain, bleeding, and bowel perforation if not treated. Patients may require long-term medication to prevent the formation of ulcers.

There may be the occurrence of post-surgical blood clots in the lungs (pulmonary embolism) or legs (deep vein thrombosis).

There may be persistent vomiting and abdominal pain.

About one-third of patients develop gallstones following a bariatric procedure. Patients must be given supplemental bile salts for at least six months following surgery.

Nutritional deficiencies such as anemia, osteoporosis, and metabolic bone disease can occur.

Regular intake of vitamins and mineral supplements must be ensured to avoid this.

Strictures or narrowing can occur at the site of the surgical anastomoses.

Bleeding and infection can occur at the laparoscopic insertion sites.

Reactive hypoglycemia can occur six months after the procedure.

Frankly, if I was a bariatric patient, I would not care about the complications! If I continued to be overweight and ill, I would suffer from the complications of obesity. The average complication rate in bariatric surgery is between four percent and seven percent, and the risk of death from surgery is one percent.

But this is the same as the complication rates related to several surgeries like the cesarian section and laparoscopic cholecystectomy surgery! However, the rate of complications with untreated obesity could well be in the range of 80 percent to 90 percent.

## Ideal Candidate for Bariatric Surgery

The Obesity and Metabolic Surgery Society of India (OSSI) has given clear guidelines for the criteria to be followed while selecting patients to undergo bariatric weight-loss surgeries.[5] Patient with a BMI above 37.5 without any obesity-related health problems or comorbidities.

Patient with a BMI above 32.5 with concomitant type 2 diabetes or any other obesity-related comorbidity. This includes conditions such as type 2 diabetes mellitus, hypertension, sleep apnea, non-alcoholic fatty liver disease, osteoarthritis, lipid abnormalities, and heart diseases. Patients should have undergone counseling and must be committed to losing weight and ready for long-term follow-up.

Other conservative methods of weight loss should have been attempted and failed. This includes having tried a definitive weight loss program that included diet, exercise, and lifestyle changes.

Patients who are considered for bariatric surgery must be in the age group of 18 to 65 years.

Patients over 65 years of age may be considered for bariatric surgery if they have very severe obesity-related comorbidities.

Bariatric surgery is also considered in patients below 18 years in certain special situations following pediatric and endocrine assessment to ensure puberty and completion of skeletal maturity.

Contraindications for Bariatric Surgery. Bariatric surgery is not recommended for patients with the following conditions:

Inflammatory diseases, such as Crohn's disease.

History of any autoimmune disease. For example, scleroderma or systemic lupus erythematosus and alcohol or drug addictions.

However, the surgeon can always make an exception on a case-to-case basis.

## How would you choose your bariatric surgeon?

I started my bariatric practice in 2005. The concept was not very popular in those times and any complication related to a bariatric procedure was highlighted widely. The problem, I realized, was the mindset of the surgeons at that time. Most surgeons considered this surgery to be just another GI surgery.

This was true except for the fact that the patients who were undergoing bariatric surgery were not 'sick' in the conventional sense. They were normal people who were walking and talking normally and there was nothing wrong with them apart from having excessive weight. It is vital for surgeons to note that a complication or a misunderstanding with the preoperative or postoperative instructions can lead to extreme distress in a patient who undergoes bariatric surgery. I remember a colleague of mine who performed a bariatric procedure on a healthcare worker without telling her that it would reduce the amount of food that she could consume after surgery. Post-surgery, she wrote him hate mails for four years.

That is why preoperative counseling is extremely important for those contemplating bariatric surgery and adequate time should be given to the prospective patients to understand and absorb what he/she will be undergoing and how it will affect their day-to-day life.

Complications following bariatric surgery can be minimized if adequate measures are taken preoperatively in patient selection, patient education and counseling, assessment of patient motivation, selection of an experienced surgeon, and selection of the most suitable bariatric procedure for the particular patient. As I figured out in my days at the Mayo Clinic, care needs to be taken that bariatric surgery is offered only to those patients who fit into the candidate criteria outlined for the procedure. Patients should be offered adequate counseling and must be educated about the surgical procedure, the benefits of the surgery, potential complications, and side effects. They must be made aware and must be willing to make the necessary changes to their diet and their lifestyle.

The importance of following a regular exercise program should be stressed and the patient must agree to do the same. The patients must be given enough time to understand and think over the drastic changes they need to make. Patients who are at a high risk of developing complications should not be offered surgery immediately; instead, they should be primed and optimized for the procedure. Bariatric surgery should not be considered an option for those having a limited life expectancy. General suitability to undergo a surgical procedure must be assessed. In India, not many healthcare centers have the volume (number of patients undergoing bariatric procedures) that a typical US center would have; so choose wisely. Choose a bariatric center that has a record of performing successful procedures with a minimal complication rate. A multidisciplinary team should be involved in the procedure. The team should have experienced surgeons, nurses, physiotherapists, dieticians, gastroenterologists, and counselors. All these professionals should be trained specifically in bariatric surgical procedures and the care of patients who have undergone the same.

The dietician, for example, should be competent to provide the right dietary guidance peculiar to a post-bariatric surgery patient. Adequate nursing care is very important in the early recognition and avoiding of complications like deep vein thrombosis and infections. The patient must be encouraged for early ambulation.

Dietary care: The dietary aspect plays the most important role in the success of the bariatric procedure. The patients must be informed about the right foods that they need to consume and the correct quantity as well. Supplements must be provided as required to avoid postoperative mineral and vitamin deficiencies. Adequate intake of protein must be ensured. Reactive hypoglycemia should be managed with dietary modifications, such as restricting carbohydrate intake and avoiding fast-acting carbohydrates.

Guidance and counseling are integral parts of the procedure and should be readily available to the patients, especially regarding lifestyle changes, to help the patients stay motivated.

Assessment of the general health of the patient should be made on a regular basis and issues such as flabby skin must be addressed. Patients may need cosmetic surgery after about a year and a half to get the right contours. Patients may require medications for reducing gastric acid secretions.

Annual laboratory tests are usually done to assess the nutritional status of the patient and address any deficiencies.

For example, Hb, blood picture, and serum ferritin to rule out anemia, serum creatinine, serum albumin to assess protein intake, vitamin levels, and plasma glucose or HbA1C.

Bone density and Vitamin D levels must be measured, especially in those undergoing gastric bypass surgery, to avoid osteoporosis.

**Who can perform bariatric surgery?**

In India, for the most part, bariatric surgical procedures are unregulated. Basically, this means that any surgeon trained in abdominal surgical procedures can undertake to perform bariatric surgical procedures as well.

The exact qualifications necessary have not been clearly spelled out. There is no specific mandatory accreditation for performing bariatric surgical procedures.

## Why has bariatric surgery not gained popularity in India?

Bariatric surgery never gained traction in India because of a lot of patient dissatisfaction. While most people would have heard of the procedure in our country, on further questioning you are likely to find that most of them hold a negative view toward the surgery and consider it potentially dangerous. This is the result of a lack of understanding of the procedure and a good dose of negative publicity highlighting the complications.

At present, statistics report that around 40,000 bariatric procedures are performed per year in India, whereas in the U.S., around 200,000 surgeries are performed per year. This is a very small number for India considering that the Indian population is around five times that of the U.S.

There are a number of morbidly obese patients in our country with severe comorbidities such as hypertension, diabetes, sleep apnea, etc. All these patients are in need of weight-loss surgery and can benefit greatly from it.

In fact, the OSSI guidelines specify lower BMI criteria for bariatric surgery than the guidelines in Western Countries do. This is due to our smaller build and the earlier occurrence of obesity-related complications when compared to that of our Western counterparts. India is a nation with limited medical resources. Bariatric surgery prevents complications from ever happening and burdening the system further. Despite the reduction in the BMI criteria for Indians, not many patients are willing to undergo this procedure. My Mayo experience taught me a few valuable things, where all patients underwent sufficient screening before being considered as candidates for bariatric surgery.

The following issues were looked into:

Has the patient made other attempts at losing weight? How many attempts did he/she make and what methods were tried?

Is the patient aware of the actual procedure? Is the patient psychologically prepared? Has he/she been informed of the lifestyle and dietary changes that would be required?

Has the patient been given sufficient time to assimilate all this information and make an informed decision? Is the patient ready for the new life he/she would face and the constant follow-up required in the initial 6 to 18 months?

From this, it is evident that the overall patient experience in the West was tremendously different from that in India. In my opinion, although the surgeons in India were extremely skillful and were able to perform bariatric procedures with competence, there was a compromise of long-term patient satisfaction because of a lack of detailed preoperative workup and patient counseling. It, therefore, followed that the patients who underwent these surgeries initially had a very skewed idea of the procedure and the results that could be achieved. The overall effect of this was the accumulation of a huge number of dissatisfied patients.

The surgeons too were unaware of the importance of preoperative measures that were needed before patients could accept this kind of surgery. Patients were pushed into accepting procedures for which they were mentally unprepared. The result of this was the loss of word-of-mouth and the specialty, unfortunately, suffered a bad name. Everyone considered bariatric surgery to be a magical solution or cure to obesity and it was promoted that way. Patients presumed they would be able to lose all their excess weight without any effort on their part. However, the reality is quite different. Bariatric surgery is only a tool that can aid in weight loss. And just like any other tool, it comes with its own set of instructions and guidelines.

You will be able to use the tool effectively only when you have understood the instructions provided clearly and abide by them. If you attempt to use it without understanding the instructions or without paying heed to them, you are only liable to hurt yourself.

**Present Day Scenario:**

Things have changed quite a lot since the early days of bariatric surgery. Now, surgeons and patients have a better understanding of how bariatric surgery works. There are many excellent centers in India offering bariatric surgery for weight loss that provide exemplary care to the patients. Some of these centers can easily beat any of those from the West with regard to results of surgery and patient satisfaction. Surgeons too are now conscious of the fact that bariatric surgical procedures are not the same as the other run-of-the-mill gastrointestinal surgeries.

Here, the patient profile is different. The postoperative implications are different. And lastly, the follow-up and lifestyle changes required are different. These patients cannot withstand complications of surgery as well as those undergoing other GI tract surgeries. Therefore, maximum care must be taken to avoid or minimize postoperative complications. In fact, during my training in the U.S., one of my professors used to say,

"When I perform a bariatric surgical procedure, it means I am actually married to the patient for about 18 months." That is the level of postoperative hand-holding and follow-up care that is required.

The 18-month postoperative period is crucial because this is the time when the patient experiences maximum weight loss and also the time when most of the complications show up. The surgeon and his team must be prepared to address all these issues.

It is likely that over time, the surgeons who were already performing these procedures will give up and stop doing them as they did not get the expected result of a happy and satisfied patient. Many of their patients will probably return with post-procedure weight gain as well. There will be newer surgeons to take their place who are more aware and informed. They will approach the whole situation with the right outlook and preparation.

### What should you look for?

Competent surgeons trained under an expert. Accredited centers where these surgeries are undertaken as a routine. These are the centers that have well-oiled machinery to deal with all kinds of scenarios.

Facilities for preoperative and postoperative counseling and follow-up care should be in place. Psychological support must be accessible to the patient.

The Red flags:

Your surgeon proposes surgery the next day. Your surgeon does not have a ready team to assess your issues preoperatively. Your surgeon proposes to cut down the cost of the surgery steeply (he looks desperate to operate). Your surgeon does not discuss the complications of the procedure freely with you or avoids answering your questions.

Solution: STAY AWAY and seek another opinion.

| Values | Credits | Surgeon A | Surgeon B | Surgeon C | Surgeon D | Surgeon E |
|---|---|---|---|---|---|---|
| Education | 1-4 | | | | | |
| Experience | 1-3 | | | | | |
| Availability | 1-3 | | | | | |
| Behavior | 1-3 | | | | | |
| Personality | 1-2 | | | | | |
| Word of mouth | 1-4 | | | | | |
| Internet likes | 1-2 | | | | | |
| Ikigai | 1-3 | | | | | |
| Testimonials | 1-2 | | | | | |
| Video-Testimonials | 1-4 | | | | | |
| Total | | | | | | |

# 8
# THE CENTRE OF THE
# BEGINNING OF A FAMILY
## Obstetrics And Gynaecology

*"Apprehension, uncertainty, waiting, expectation, fear of surprise, do a patient more harm than any exertion."* – Florence Nightingale

Gynaecologists are specialists who focus on the female reproductive organs and the diseases that affect them. Obstetrics on the other hand involves pregnancy and delivery, menstruation, and reproductive concerns, while sexually transmitted infections (STIs), hormone imbalances, and other issues are all dealt with by either of them. Together they are known as the Department of Obstetrics and Gynaecology. We will elaborate on their areas of care as we progress into the chapter. Women begin going for a consultation to the obstetrics and gynaecology department in their early adolescence and continue to attend a well-woman clinic for general health concerns. Women usually visit their gynaecologist (also known as the women's specialist) at least once a year for a checkup or whenever they have any symptoms that worry them.

Yes! women make up almost half the population on earth.

Obstetricians and gynaecologists are typically consulted for all issues relating to menstruation, pregnancy, infertility, contraception, pregnancy termination where indicated, menopause, diseases of the pelvic organs, and disorders affecting the ligaments and muscles that support the pelvic organs. They also treat patients with polycystic ovarian syndrome (PCOS), vulvar and vaginal ulcers, gynaecological cancers, and other non-cancerous dysplasia, as well as premalignant conditions, such as endometrial hyperplasia and cervical dysplasia. While the obstetricians attend emergencies like delivering babies who decide to come anytime, caesarian sections, and ectopic pregnancies (these can rupture and give way to massive bleeds that can become life-threatening), the gynaecologists have their own set of emergency issues to take care of.

Congenital anomalies of the female reproductive tract; endometriosis, a chronic illness that affects the reproductive system; and pelvic inflammatory disorders, such as abscesses are some of the other conditions for which they are consulted. Some of them could be life-threatening, such as ovarian torsion or a ruptured ovarian cyst.

What happens in the doctor's office is determined by the cause for the visit as well as the circumstances of the individual. So, how do you decide whom to see in case of an issue pertaining to the female reproductive system? To start with, all the students who take up the branch, are trained in obstetrics and gynaecology; however, after a few years, a few of them would leave obstetrics and focus only on gynaecology or vice versa, or a few would leave both and just focus on gynaecological malignancy or infertility. When it comes to gynaecology, it can be said that it is far more structured than the world of surgeons. They do not possess a higher specialised degree other than the basic MS degree in Obstetrics and Gynaecology. If they want to get noticed quickly, they will need to invest in extra training. When a typical gynaecologist graduates, he or she will be able to handle a normal delivery, perform caesarian sections, and comprehend the complications associated with childbirth.

India is a huge country, and it has a large population and high birth rates; as a result, a regular government hospital-trained gynaecologist would be able to successfully perform normal deliveries and caesarean sections as a routine, right from day one after they graduate. Gynaecologists would not need to do much to get started in their careers; they could just get attached to a nursing home and attract a large number of patients. As previously mentioned, the gynaecological practice may be separated into two categories: 'Obstetrics' and 'Gynaecology'. The obstetric practice or obstetrics basically deals with the care of pregnant women, the unborn baby, and childbirth—labor and delivery. The obstetrician ensures that the patient has a safe pregnancy throughout what is called the antenatal period, a safe delivery, and a safe postnatal period where certain complications may occur, such as excessive bleeding and infections.

Gynaecologists, on the other hand, deal with all other ailments involving the female reproductive system. Women remain under the gynaecologist's care in all stages of their life, right from puberty, also known as menarche, until menopause and beyond as well. Let us look at the practice of gynaecology and obstetrics independently at first, and then study the sub-specialties within the system. Patients may have a normal delivery or a caesarean section and this depends on the progress of labor, and other indications, such as foetal distress. Caesarean sections are sometimes performed as elective procedures in certain conditions where it is unsafe for the baby or the mother to undergo normal delivery. This is the standard obstetric practice. However, there is a minor issue with this. The obstetric practice grows more labor intense as one becomes older and as the surgeon's practice grows. The precise time a patient will go into labor is unknown. And when it does happen, it is akin to a medical emergency in which one must ensure that both the baby and the mother are in good health: the baby must not be in respiratory distress, because this can result in complications like aspiration of the amniotic fluid, failing to breathe on being born, or worse, stillbirth.

The practice of obstetrics, as you can see, is fraught with stress and anxiety.

Now, if you look at a typical practice of the 'Gynaecology' speciality, it usually would start with an obstetric practice.

An obstetric practice would have a female patient with a pregnancy interacting with a doctor, who would then hold her hand for the next nine months. This occurs right after conception when the patient misses her periods for the first time. At this point in time, the gynaecologist would be highly concerned with what is going on with her, such as her blood pressure, diabetes status, and the position of the baby throughout the pregnancy. Well, it probably is a very busy practice. So then, at the end of the nine months, it culminates in a delivery, which could be a normal one or a caesarean section. There are many more conditions that the obstetrician needs to watch out for. This kind of practice requires a very energetic gynaecologist. A baby does not care if the gynaecologist is in a meeting or having dinner or is at a party.

When the baby decides to arrive, born it will be, and the doctor will have to drop whatever he/she is doing and rush to the hospital. These days, a new development is the birthing suite, where a mom can have her baby under relaxed conditions as opposed to the old way of delivering in a labor room, which has a distinct clinical atmosphere. The in-thing now is to pamper the mother with a relaxed soothing atmosphere, so that the whole birthing experience is enjoyable.

All pregnancy-related issues, the birth, and the baby are well taken care of. The usual scenario is this: The gynaecologist who cared for your mother is probably now in her 60s. Her practice is more of gynaecology than obstetrics. The baby she delivered is now pregnant herself! That is the second generation for her. The experience is invaluable. Getting the correct input or advice for your condition is very important. A gynaecologist becomes famous based on the kind of practice that he/she establishes in the initial years.

It requires a lot of empathy and a lot of hours missed away from the home. As gynaecologists grow older, they begin to wonder if it is worth their while to leave their family and friends to attend a single delivery when the baby would be born anyway.

Today, with litigations being so common, any normal delivery has the potential to turn into a very precarious one where an urgent surgical intervention in the form of a caesarean section is indicated. This is the point where the gynaecologist starts introspecting. They begin to wonder if it is worth the effort and time and sacrifice on their part. They try to find peace and a practice that is more comfortable for them, where they can keep to their own timings, come and go in their own timings.

This is the point where most of the gynaecologists start to develop teams where the younger doctors would attend to the normal deliveries. However, in a complicated case or when decisions and crucial diagnoses have to be made, the seniors would take the responsibility. All caesarean sections are usually performed by the senior gynaecologist.

This is the period when the gynaecologists start restricting themselves to gynaecological practice and surgeries only, after many years of going through sleepless nights. In my practice, I have seen a lot of gynaecologists who continue to do obstetric practice well into their senior years just because they enjoy their work. As we progress further into the 21st century, more and more gynaecologists will abandon the practice of obstetrics and only practice gynaecology, though this will require specialised training after their postgraduate degrees and they may be required to work under someone for a period of time to gain experience.

However, as a surgeon, one will have a better life and be able to achieve a better work-life balance, as well as have the benefit of not having to hurry in the middle of the night for an obstetrics case.

So, this practice also involves the gynaecologist getting trained in newer procedures like 'laparoscopic surgery.' The majority of procedures involving the uterus and ovaries may be performed laparoscopically, which means through a small incision.

Laparoscopic surgery offers several significant advantages compared to regular surgery. As it involves smaller incisions, there is less bleeding, less pain, wound healing is faster, and there is a shorter hospital stay required.

Moreover, there is less discomfort associated with scar healing and one can resume their normal physical activities much sooner than they would have with a regular open abdomen surgery. In laparoscopic surgery, manipulation of the organs is minimal, and this possibly results in less internal scarring as well. Traditional procedures may need you to stay in the hospital for a week or longer, with a total recovery time of four to eight weeks. If you undergo laparoscopic surgery, you may only need to stay in the hospital for two nights and recuperate in two or three weeks. In addition, a shorter hospital stay is usually less expensive. You might have been diagnosed with an ovarian or uterine cyst or some other condition requiring a hysterectomy, that is the removal of the uterus.

Some doctors might tell you that the best approach to remove the uterus or ovaries would be via an open surgery, which would involve making an incision in the lower abdominal region and removing the uterus and the ovaries.

However, most gynaecologists now believe that this is not the ideal method and that the best way to remove the cyst is through a keyhole surgery. In earlier times, there were not many gynaecologists who were trained to perform laparoscopic surgeries, and this was the dilemma. These operations were then performed by general surgeons who had the necessary expertise and training and were skilled in laparoscopic surgery. However, as time went on, an increasing number of gynaecologists became quite comfortable performing laparoscopic operations and were able to perform laparoscopic gynaecological surgeries. Now, these gynaecologists who have the required training and expertise in laparoscopic surgery hold a super-specialised position; it is no surprise that they are the ones who are increasingly less concerned with obstetrics. Uterine fibroid is one of the conditions where laparoscopic surgery is indicated.

These benign tumours of the uterus are highly prevalent, with 35 percent to 60 percent of women developing them by the age of 35, and 70 percent to 80 percent by the age of 50. Excessive uterine bleeding, infertility, and miscarriages are all symptoms of uterine fibroids.

A traditional hysterectomy (the removal of the uterus to remove fibroids) through an incision in the lower abdomen usually involves a five-day stay in the hospital.

Getting referrals from your trusted family doctor, friends, or relatives is the first and most important step in finding the correct gynaecologist or obstetrician.

Take your time to look into the credentials, experience, and skills of the gynaecologist. If the gynaecologist makes you feel at ease, you can discuss your concerns with him or her.

It is crucial that they have an approachable demeanour and a receptive mindset. The doctor should be willing to engage in a two-way dialogue and answer any questions you might have. If you have a complicated gynaecological condition or are pregnant with a high-risk pregnancy, you may require the services of a skilled gynaecologist/obstetrician as a few centres now specialise in high-risk pregnancies. As a patient, it is critical to understand the differences between the various types of obstetric practices. For example, if you choose a senior gynaecologist, they would probably have a team under them performing both gynae and obstetric procedures.

Most likely, the birthing will be overseen by a young doctor working under the senior gynaecologist. The senior doctor may not be able to give you enough time to clear all your doubts, although I doubt that the final outcomes may differ in different situations. If this situation is acceptable to you, then you may select a senior gynaecologist.

However, if you are concerned about personalised care, you should seek someone who can be kind to you during your pregnancy, look after you well, and give you sound advice in terms of your personal and emotional life.

This should be someone who can provide you with a clear idea of what to expect during these times and the many surgical and nonsurgical treatments available to you. Basically, you would become comfortable with your obstetrician through the antenatal period and the rest of the journey through labor and childbirth would be easy. So, if you are with a gynaecologist with 10 to 20 years of experience and you are looking for an obstetric service,

I believe those are the people who are best suited to care for you for your obstetric needs. They would be young, energetic, and available!

If it is a gynaecology practice, the senior the gynaecologist, the better it is for you, because a senior person will be able to understand your needs and advice you on what is best for you: Is a hysterectomy indicated? Or should the uterus be preserved? How should the ovarian cyst be treated? And much more.

One of the offshoots of the Gynae/Obs. practice is the treatment for infertility. It has now become a branch in itself and many young postgraduates take up advanced courses in infertility management and pursue it as a super-specialisation. The advances in the infertility space are mind-boggling. Test tube babies and surrogacy are in demand as more and more women are concerned about their looks post-pregnancy.

Most in-vitro fertilisation (IVF) labs have state-of-the-art technology, such as laser hatching, and experts handling the IVF procedures.

Finding an infertility expert is pretty straightforward. Choose the lab and the doctor with maximum success rates. The net is filled with credentials that can be verified through a phone call or an e-mail. What is ironic about the infertility practice is that, although the treatment is very logical like mathematics, the result is not! Typically, it is very easy to find out what the problem is with the couple and this is logical like maths, but when the treatment is administered to two couples who have exactly the same problem, the outcomes may be vastly different. We try to be Gods, but we are not!

Another area where obstetricians and gynaecologists have a role to play and one that is emerging at a rapid pace is gynae malignancies. Gynae oncology is an upcoming branch that deals with cancers of the female reproductive system.

Although surgeries on the breast for cancer or other related problems do not come under gynaecology, many experienced gynae consultants are equally capable of handling them and so are the onco-surgeons, who have an MCh degree in oncosurgery.

The reason why gynaecological malignancies are distinct and require specialist treatment is that while cancer care surgeons may be able to do a wonderful job for cancer patients, an onco-gynaecologist will be able to look at the aesthetics apart from the good clearance of the tumour as they are well versed in that area of anatomy as well and will be able to do an equally good job. A large number of gynaecological cancer specialists are currently doing robotic procedures.

They are using robots to perform onco-gynaecological surgeries. They have also been taught how to perform the same procedures laparoscopically. However, the choice of the procedure depends on the surgeon as well as the patient: Which procedure does the surgeon think will benefit the patient more? What procedure does the patient wish to undergo? Can the patient afford to undergo a robotic procedure? Personally, I believe that robotic surgery in the pelvis has got significant advantages compared to conventional laparoscopic surgeries.

If someone is diagnosed with a gynaecological cancer, I would advise you to explore your choices. Obtain many opinions in order to determine the precise diagnosis of your condition, and if it is malignancy, you should seek treatment from a professional who is doing the procedure as a routine. Your family gynaecologist could be the first person you contact. I doubt that any of them would provide you with bad counsel. Even if they ask you to be admitted, and they are not too sure of your case, chances are he/she will make sure that an expert is investigating your case.

So, at the end of the day, I would advise you to follow your heart and take informed decisions.

Therefore, it is vital that you maintain your relationship with your family gynaecologist, who can guide you even if she herself is not performing laparoscopic/robotic surgeries.

I have mentioned before that the organs present in the female pelvis, such as the ovaries, the fallopian tubes, and the uterus and cervix, can be approached laparoscopically. Unfortunately, surgeons belonging to the older generation are not typically comfortable with laparoscopic procedures.

In the last ten years, a large number of young gynaecologists have begun doing laparoscopic operations, with great outcomes. The same procedures can now be performed robotically as well, using smaller incisions with the surgeon sitting and performing the procedure via a robot.

There is a very significant cost difference between laparoscopic and robotic procedures, with the cost being much higher for the latter. Owing to this reason, presently, cancer procedures are the most common indication for robotic surgery. In an obstetric practice, the situation is pretty straightforward. Both the patients and doctors have a choice. If the patient is comfortable with having an older surgeon operate on them, then they would do so. Or the gynaecologists can call in younger, well-trained laparoscopic surgeons who can operate on their behalf, under their supervision.

Well, the bottom line here is decision-making. What is the diagnosis and what would be the right treatment? That is the KEY. I would say decision-making by an older experienced gynaecologist or surgeon will definitely be better for you than decisions made by a younger less-experienced gynaecologist.

| Values | Credits | Surgeon A | Surgeon B | Surgeon C | Surgeon D | Surgeon E |
|---|---|---|---|---|---|---|
| Education | 1-4 | | | | | |
| Experience | 1-3 | | | | | |
| Availability | 1-3 | | | | | |
| Behavior | 1-3 | | | | | |
| Personality | 1-2 | | | | | |
| Word of mouth | 1-4 | | | | | |
| Internet likes | 1-2 | | | | | |
| Ikigai | 1-3 | | | | | |
| Testimonials | 1-2 | | | | | |
| Video-Testimonials | 1-4 | | | | | |
| Total | | | | | | |

# 9

# WE FIX THE LEAKS
## Urology

*"Health care historically has been a very siloed field that's organized around medical specialties - urology, cardiac surgery, and so forth - and around the supply of these specialty services. The patient is the ping-pong ball that moves from service to service."* - Michael Porter

When it comes to diseases involving the urinary tract, choosing the super-specialty for consultation is quite straightforward—You would visit the urologist.

The guys that do the job are awesome, and most importantly, they are a happy lot! (Happiness quotient is just next to that of the Orthopaedicians). The field of urology covers conditions involving the male and female urinary systems and the male reproductive organs. A specialist qualifies to become a urologist after completing his/her Master's in General Surgery followed by the MCh. degree in Urology. Anything from a prostate problem to kidney stones is dealt with by the urologists.

If you are experiencing difficulty passing urine or you have been diagnosed with cancer of the bladder, kidneys, or ureters, you would have to see a urologist.

It appears that your options are limited and uncomplicated when it comes to the specialty of Urology. The close proximity of all the organs making up the genitourinary system in the pelvis makes any surgical intervention on these really tricky. Urinary tract injuries in women can commonly occur during gynaecological surgeries. Urinary tract damage is estimated to account for 0.2%–1% of all gynaecologic and pelvic surgeries. A qualified urologist is the best person to sort out these cases. Injuries to the urinary system in women caused by obstetric and gynaecologic operations are usually divided into two categories: Acute problems, such as bladder or ureteric damage, can be detected and corrected during the procedure, while chronic consequences, such as vesicovaginal fistula (VVF) and ureterovaginal fistula (UVF), might appear days to months following the primary surgery. Ninety percent of these fistulas occur in impoverished nations, particularly India, as a result of neglected and obstructed childbirth. Urologists are increasingly doing complex, minimally invasive endoscopic and laparoscopic procedures to treat these issues.

The more expertise a urologist has in his field, the better, right? Well, that might be true, but urology is one field where you do not have to worry too much about the treatment options, which are rather clear.

Urologists seldom resort to open surgeries unless they are cancer procedures. Endoscopic techniques are used in the majority of urological surgeries.

Endoscopic operations need a high degree of skill and accuracy.

Urologists with 20 to 25 years of experience who are familiar with modern technology and can operate with minimal hand tremors may be considered the finest in their area. Although urology super-specialisation training is nearly consistent across India, when a new super-specialist doctor graduates with training in this specialty, he will be able to do at least a basic set of procedures.

These would include operations for the removal of stones from the ureters or stenting of the ureters, and a variety of other simple procedures.

They would also be trained to perform transurethral resection of the prostate (TURP) for patients requiring prostatectomy. These fundamental operations are known to be the urologist's bread and butter, but when it comes to complexities resulting from post-operative complications, an experienced urologist is needed.

Now, many of those urology patients who undergo TURP, a procedure usually performed in older men for urinary problems, may experience either difficulty in holding urine or painful urination, or they might develop a stricture of the urethra, where the surgeon was perhaps a little over-enthusiastic in his surgery and some permanent damage had been done to the urinary tract.

The commonest of these would be strictures in the urethra. This is where the urologist's experience comes into play; an experienced urologist will know just how much to cut. As a result, the patients are quite comfortable postoperatively.

They do not develop any problems in passing urine or any other complications. Experienced urologists continue to learn new surgical techniques and improve their skills as time goes by; they can perform the surgeries quicker with more accuracy, reducing anaesthesia time.

Let us now look at some of the common conditions that are treated by urologists.

Prostate hypertrophy: The commonest urological problem encountered in men is prostatic issues. Older men, especially after the age of 50, may complain of difficulty in passing urine. This is due to the enlargement of the prostate gland, which surrounds the urethra. Pressure on the urethra by the enlarged gland causes difficulties in passing urine. This condition is called Benign Prostatic Hypertrophy (BPH). Traditionally, the method used to resect the prostate gland was TURP. Now newer procedures like robotic-assisted surgery (for prostate cancer) and laser therapy (for BPH) are being used. In TURP, the urologist would put a tube in the urethra and scrape off and remove the prostatic tissue.

The laser procedure, on the other hand, is a little time-consuming, but it comes with the advantage of reduced bleeding.

So, for those patients who have cardiac conditions and are being treated with blood thinners and anti-platelet medications, laser surgery makes sense.

However, if you have no other health issues, the routine TURP procedure would work fine. The laser procedure is just bound to add to your cost. Essentially, the procedures are the same. Cancers of the urinary tract: For cancers of the bladder, kidneys, and the ureters, you should decide whether you want to consult a urologist who is competent to perform these surgeries, but is probably only performing them a couple of times in six months, or would you rather be operated on by a uro-oncologist who is trained in cancer surgery.

In my opinion, the results from the patient's health perspective may not be very different. However, the newer techniques such as robotic procedures promote faster healing and involve shorter hospital stays, and any surgeon who is trained in robotic surgery will be able to perform them. They are less painful as well, particularly in prostatic cancers. Bladder cancers can be treated by routine urological surgery or robotic procedures. The intestines are then used to make a new bladder. For kidney and ureteric cancers, the treatment is very straightforward and clear. There are guidelines in place and they have to be followed for the best results. Nephron-sparing procedures are the new surgical techniques for these malignancies.

Stones in the urinary tract: The treatment for kidney stones and ureteric stones is pretty straightforward as well. Lithotripsy and lasers are the commonly used methods for treating these conditions. The stones are broken down or crushed into smaller pieces, which can pass through the urinary tract easily. In lithotripsy, extracorporeal shock waves are used to break down the stones, whereas, in laser therapy, laser waves are used through a ureteroscope. All urologists will be trained to address these conditions competently.

As I mentioned previously, urologists seldom perform operations involving cutting open the abdomen unless it is for a cancer operation.

Urologists are the ones who usually perform cancer surgeries relating to the kidneys, the ureters, or the urinary bladder. However, I have noticed in my career that more and more individuals are now choosing to go to an oncologist surgeon who specialises in urological cancer procedures rather than to a general urologist for cancer-related operations. Uro-oncologists undergo a minimum of two years of extra training in this field in addition to their mandatory surgical and urology training.

A uro-oncologist will collaborate closely with your medical team to customise therapies to your specific malignancy and help you avoid adverse effects.

Many urologic malignancies are treated primarily with surgery. The sort of surgery required may be determined by the type and staging of the cancer.

For instance, in patients having cancer of the urinary bladder, cystectomy is performed and a new bladder is constructed out of a portion of the gastrointestinal tract. Basically, this means the entire urinary bladder is removed and a new one is fashioned out of a piece of the patient's intestine. This procedure would involve the gastrointestinal surgeons taking part as well.

Chemotherapy, radiation therapy, targeted therapy, or immunotherapy may be used if a urologic malignancy has spread. Many of the urologists are trained to perform robotic procedures as well.

Robotic surgery actually has an important role in urology because of the small area of interest, much of which lies in the pelvic cavity, which has limited accessibility. The robotic approach has a better reach and offers better manoeuvrability compared to that obtained in traditional open surgical procedures or endoscopic procedures, particularly in surgeries like Radical Prostatectomy for bladder cancer.

In the end, an experienced urologist would make a huge difference in the treatment's success.

Prostate cancer is one of the commonest malignancies in men.

ICMR has reported the incidence in India to be less than that seen in Western countries: 9–10/100,000 population.[6]

Here is some information about the diagnosis and treatment of prostate cancer.

Radical Prostatectomy is a surgery that removes the whole prostate gland. The procedure is only performed when the patient has cancer prostate. When performed using robotic surgical equipment, the results are superior to that seen with conventional prostate removal. A definitive diagnosis of cancer prostate is made after the biopsy is termed positive for cancer cells.

A prostate biopsy is a procedure where a small tissue sample of the prostate gland is removed and then looked at under a microscope.

The pathologist examines and evaluates the specimen. Endoscopic biopsies are feasible, even though most are done using image guidance, such as ultrasound, computed tomography (CT), or magnetic resonance imaging (MRI) technologies.

Radical prostatectomy is the main surgical treatment of choice. Here the entire prostate gland is resected along with some adjoining tissues. However, there are many different ways of performing a prostatectomy. Traditionally, open prostatectomy was done, but those days are long gone.

These days laparoscopic or robotic procedures have become the treatment of choice. Who would be the right person to perform this surgery: the urologist or the uro-oncologist?

The bottom line here is the person with more experience is likely to give better results for the patient. Just because a urologist is young does not mean he lacks experience.

They get better and better at their job as they get older. However, it must be mentioned that if a urologist is negligent and the patient develops a complication or an unfavourable surgical outcome, the patient ends up with a daily reminder of the same.

Bladder cancer is seen more often in men than in women. A cystoscopy is performed to examine the bladder and remove sample tissue for a biopsy. The diagnosis of cancer is based on the biopsy being positive for cancer cells. Staging of the disease is done using various imaging techniques. Depending on the stage of the disease, various surgical techniques are adopted to treat the cancer.

**Cystectomy**: Here, the entire bladder or part of the bladder is removed. When there is a single small tumor, partial cystectomy is performed, where only the portion of the bladder containing the tumor is resected. In radical cystectomy, the entire bladder is removed along with the surrounding lymph nodes as well.

In men, the prostate and seminal vesicles may be removed. In women, a portion of the vagina, the uterus, and the ovaries may be removed as part of the procedure. Radical cystectomy also entails the creation of a neobladder, which I have mentioned earlier.

**Transurethral resection of bladder tumor (TURBT)**: This procedure is used to treat those cancers that have not yet invaded the muscle layer and are restricted to the inner lining of the urinary bladder. Here, no incisions are made in the abdomen.

A cystoscope is passed through the urethra, and then either electric current or laser waves are used to burn off the cancer cells. This is a treatment for early-stage bladder malignancies.

**Robotic cystectomy**: It is a lengthy and demanding procedure. After the bladder is removed, robots are used to implant intracorporal diversions such as neobladders and ileal conduits to guarantee that urine flows freely. Compared to standard open surgery, patients who underwent this treatment experienced less blood loss, a lower transfusion rate, a shorter hospital stay, and less discomfort. Cancer of the kidney commonly occurs in the older age groups. The commonest type of kidney cancer is renal cell carcinoma. Surgical resection of the kidney depends on the extent and stage of the disease.

The entire diseased kidney is removed during radical nephrectomy. If the tumor is connected with, or extremely close to, the adrenal gland, it may also be removed. The surgeons may create incisions in the belly, beneath the ribs, or in the back to remove the whole kidney during this procedure.

**Laparoscopic radical nephrectomy (LRN)**: Instead of using one huge incision, this procedure is conducted through a series of tiny incisions. To allow the excised kidney to slide through, one of the incisions is somewhat bigger than the others. LRN may take less time to heal and result in less bleeding and scarring. Partial nephrectomy: During this treatment, the physician merely removes the cancerous portion of the kidney. Patients with cancer in both kidneys, low kidney function, or just one kidney may require this form of kidney cancer surgery to preserve kidney function. This can be termed nephron-sparing surgery.

**Testicular Cancers**: There are mainly two types of testicular cancer surgeries: The surgeon will remove the testicle with the tumor along with the spermatic cord that joins the testicle to the abdomen during a radical inguinal orchiectomy. If your doctor feels the cancer cells have moved to the surrounding lymph nodes, a retroperitoneal lymph node dissection may be performed at the same time or later during a second operation.

**Transplant Surgeries:** Although many urologists do kidney transplants, a new breed of surgeons known as transplant surgeons have emerged to take on the task of performing transplant surgeries along with urological procedures.

Compared to traditional open kidney transplant surgery, a considerably smaller incision is used in laparoscopic procedures to remove the healthy kidney from the donor and place the new kidney into the abdomen of the recipient, followed by suturing of the blood vessels and the ureter. This technique helps the otherwise healthy donor to recover from the surgery faster and painlessly.

The tools are inserted into the abdomen through small incisions. Not only do these surgeons do renal transplants, but they also perform hepatic transplants, pancreas transplants, and lung transplants.

And, for the most part, just a few urologists are still interested in doing transplants. However, there is still a ton of work available in urology that none of the other departments undertake to do as it is a highly specialised field. This is true mainly with reference to onco-surgeons as mentioned before.

None of the oncological surgeons are really interested in doing neurosurgery or urology.

**What you should know**:

When it comes to problems of routine urology, such as prostatic hypertrophy causing difficulty in urination for an elderly male, the treatment is TURP. Now you basically need to choose whether you want it done through the trans-urethral route using a cystoscope or by laser therapy. The procedure will be the same.

The only difference is whether electrocautery is used or laser waves are used. Of course, as mentioned earlier, laser therapy involves less bleeding and quicker healing. It might be the right option for patients who are on blood thinners and other cardiac medications. However, if there are no other health issues involved, the usual TURP would suffice and cost you less as well. When it comes to malignancies in the genitourinary system, you have to decide whether you want to be operated on by someone who does a minimum of these surgeries or by someone who is specially trained in these procedures and is well versed in using newer technologies such as robotic surgery.

In my opinion, there may not be much of a difference in the outcome when both surgeons are experienced, but robotic procedures can give you the benefit of being less painful with a lesser hospital stay and quicker recovery. This is especially true for prostatic tumors and bladder malignancies.

Bladder cancers will involve open surgeries when advanced, and these may be performed by the urologist quite competently. Surgeons from other specialties might be called in as well. However, the advantage of going to an oncological urologist is that they would be competent in the entire cancer protocol.

Kidney malignancies require just a resection of the entire kidney, which can be performed by a urologist. However, when the cancer is not advanced, patients are now being offered partial nephrectomy or nephron-sparing procedures.

In advanced cases, where the surrounding structures are affected as well, vascular surgeons, gastrointestinal surgeons, and cardiothoracic surgeons might need to assist the urologist.

For stones in the urinary tract, it is really very straightforward. All urologists are trained to deal with them and it is really a no-brainer.

The bottom line is that if you have sufficient funds, you may go in for laser surgery and robotic procedures. If you do not have the funds, the regular endoscopic procedures are good enough. The only difference is a small increase in morbidity and a little longer stay in the hospital.

So, if you can afford it, be a bit courageous and give yourself a little advantage.

# INCISIONS

| Values | Credits | Surgeon A | Surgeon B | Surgeon C | Surgeon D | Surgeon E |
|---|---|---|---|---|---|---|
| Education | 1-4 | | | | | |
| Experience | 1-3 | | | | | |
| Availability | 1-3 | | | | | |
| Behavior | 1-3 | | | | | |
| Personality | 1-2 | | | | | |
| Word of mouth | 1-4 | | | | | |
| Internet likes | 1-2 | | | | | |
| Ikigai | 1-3 | | | | | |
| Testimonials | 1-2 | | | | | |
| Video-Testimonials | 1-4 | | | | | |
| Total | | | | | | |

# 10
# THE BONES!
## Orthopedics

The happiest guys in the hospitals are the orthopaedic surgeons!

No matter what, they remain happy and the other guys have no idea why! They might be competent surgeons in their field, but if you ask them to move just a wee bit outside their territory or field, they just do not care.

They will be happy to operate on a patient whose haemoglobin level is just 8 gm%, while their anaesthetist would blow his top! The only criterion they consider is whether the patient is willing to take the risk! There are tons of jokes about orthopaedic surgeons, and let me tell you, they just do not care! There is a joke that was very popular around the time we graduated.

The story goes that an orthopaedic surgeon was running late and rushed into the hospital. As he ran into the lobby, he saw the elevator doors closing. He found the energy to sprint and stuck his head between the closing doors. The doors crashed into his head and opened as they met with an obstruction.

He stepped into the elevator to the shock of those already inside. The orthopaedic surgeon began to rub and massage his head, which had received quite a nasty blow.

One of the other passengers on the elevator could not help but ask, "Why didn't you use your hands to stop the doors?" The orthopaedic surgeon looked incredulously at the questioner and answered, "I am an orthopaedic surgeon and I need my hands for my work."

During my training, there used to be a saying that the orthopaedic surgeon led a life of luxury and had to only show up whenever there were fractures involved. If you have knee joint pain, you could get a joint replacement, which can be expensive and thus be a luxury. The joint pain per se is not likely to kill you, except maybe if you overdose on pain killers. My mother-in-law suffered from severe knee joint pain. Even today, at the age of 85, she has a limp due to her ailment. However, she does not feel that undergoing joint replacement surgery is an urgent need. She has lost a lot of weight and is able to walk around without great discomfort. If she had had a fall, in the olden days, the treatment procedure would have been quite elaborate. She would have been encased in plaster of Paris and put in traction. Essentially, fractures in the earlier days were treated by putting the affected body part in a cast and prescribing a long period of bed rest for the patient; this would inevitably lead to the other complications of prolonged bed rest, such as bed sores. Perhaps, the mistaken idea that the specialty of orthopaedics only dealt with fractures gained much prevalence due to these casts. However, if you trace the history of orthopaedics, you will be surprised.

It has undergone significant evolution over time, especially in the past two decades. In this period, the orthopaedic department has moved from being perceived as a luxury department to an urgent and necessary branch of medicine. This statement brings forth two fundamental questions which need to be answered. What can be considered a luxury? And what can be considered a necessity?

I got a joint replacement done for my mother when she was 80 years old. It was not an easy decision to take.

My mother was skeptical, and so was I. We were not sure of the effectiveness of such a procedure, especially at her age. However, one person was not skeptical. It was her orthopaedic surgeon.

He was confident and reassured us that there would not be any problems. We took him at his word and the surgery went forward without a hitch. There was a three-month rehabilitation program to help my mother get used to the new joints. After the three-month program, she was able to adjust to life very quickly.

She was able to function properly without any issues. Six months after her surgery, my father fell ill. He was diagnosed to have cancer. My mother was able to look after both my father and herself for the next year without any assistance. Just imagine the scenario if she had not undergone the surgery. She would still be suffering from joint pain and would not have been able to walk. I can only imagine the pain and guilt she would have felt in that case. Her quality of life would have been severely affected if she had to take care of her husband while she struggled to walk.

An 84-year-old neighbor slipped and fell in the shower damaging her hip joint. The treatment at one time would have been traction and a long period of bed rest.

She wanted to get back on her feet quickly. She, too, opted for surgery. Her hip joint was fixed within a day. She was able to walk within three or four days. If any person meets her today, they will never even know that she had undergone a hip joint replacement. I can say that from experience. When I met her one-and-half years after the operation, she walked with a tiny limp. If I were not aware of the fact, I would never have guessed that she had undergone a hip joint replacement.

In the present times, the orthopaedic department treats most of the common ailments promptly. If anyone suffers from a fracture, they are immediately operated upon. The plating, stenting, pins, and screws are brought to use very quickly if needed. This is extremely important to ensure that there is no drop in the quality of life after patients recover from their injuries and ailments. This brings us to the decision of choosing an orthopaedic surgeon.

When you sustain a fracture, you do not have the luxury of time to question and decide on your surgeon. Thus, the best choice would be to check the orthopaedics department in any big, clean reputed hospital.

Just check for one thing. Are the premises of the department kept clean? If the department places importance on cleanliness and orderliness, you can trust the surgeons within that department.

If you are operated on for any fractures, even if a plate has been pinned and screwed on for treatment, you will most likely be able to do light walking in three to four days and go home.

The images of patients in big casts in hospital beds with their affected leg in a splint can be consigned to movies of old. You may presume that only a good orthopaedic surgeon can perform such procedures. However, that is not true; any general orthopaedician will be able to accomplish this task.

The quality of an orthopaedic surgeon only comes into play when the treatments are a bit more complicated, for example, if there is any reconstruction work. Reconstructive surgery is an offshoot of orthopaedic surgery. It requires the skill and patience of the surgeon. It involves tasks that can be repetitive and it can be physically demanding. Reconstructive procedures are highly challenging and can place extreme strain on the operating surgeon, even to the extent of damaging their musculoskeletal system.[7] This study looked at the prevalence of work-related injuries among orthopaedic surgeons who specialised in adult reconstructive surgery. As per this study, 66.1 percent of the surgeons surveyed suffered from an injury due to these challenging operations that they routinely performed.

The most common injuries were lower back pain, shoulder tendonitis, lumbar disc herniation, lateral epicondylitis of the elbow, and wrist arthritis. The study also reported that 27 percent of the surgeons had to take time off due to their injuries and 31 percent of the surgeons also needed surgery to treat their injuries.

Joint reconstruction differs from joint replacement.

In the former, the surgeon will be trying to salvage a joint by preserving as much natural bone and tissue as possible. It requires great expertise and skill on the part of the surgeon to carry out this procedure. Joint replacement, on the other hand, involves the removal of a damaged joint and replacing it with an entirely new joint made out of man-made components. The efficacy and success of either of these procedures depend entirely upon the skill of the surgeon.

I am of the firm belief that it is the surgeon's skill that determines the degree of improvement. One way to identify a good surgeon for a particular operation or procedure is to find the number of times the surgeon has performed the said procedure. But if you are looking for an orthopaedic surgeon to perform either a joint reconstruction or joint replacement surgery, you will have to look beyond the raw numbers. Let us assume a surgeon conducts five or six joint operations in a day. It may seem impressive, but in such cases, the surgeon will not be performing the whole surgery, and neither should you expect him to do so. The key parts in these surgeries determine the success of the procedure and that is where he would step in once the other initial steps are taken care of. Such surgeons have well-trained assistants who are well-attuned to the surgeon's methods. The assistants will do the cutting, scraping, and suturing. The surgeon will perform the important tasks like putting the joint in place and then move on to the next operation. In the grand scheme of things, the surgeon may only be doing the minimum work.

However, the surgeon is assigned the most critical tasks because he has to conserve his physical and mental energy, especially when he has to deal with a number of procedures in a day. If the surgeon is between 50 and 60 years of age, it will be practically impossible to perform six to seven surgeries per day and do a good job in all of them. The study that I referenced earlier also points out that the time-off required for surgeons increased when they were over the age of 55 and had been in practice for more than 20 years.

So, the assistants or associates do the lion's share of the work and leave the critical parts of the surgery to the senior surgeon.

The surgeon performs the critical part as your mobility and pain relief depend on that part.

*"A good assistant does not always become a good chief, but a bad assistant never does. A good chief has always been a good assistant."* – Charles FM Saint

Another key area that has developed under orthopaedic surgery has been sports medicine. There might be a perception that sports medicine is related to the treatment of superstar athletes. It was even in the news recently when the Board of Control for Cricket in India (BCCI) announced that it was planning to start a sports medicine research facility in its upcoming Centre for Excellence in Bangalore. In a bid to make it a fertile ground for sports medicine research, the BCCI held talks with medical research institutes and universities. It also planned to create a sports medicine curriculum and upgrade the qualification criteria for physios and trainers.[8] When one reads news articles like the above, it is understandable to think that sports medicine is an offshoot of orthopaedics that caters to high-performance athletes. However, it is understood differently, especially in the West. It is indeed a specialty and offshoot of orthopaedics. However, the mistaken assumption comes from the understanding of the word sports. The term 'sports' referred to here is not just about superstar athletes. It is about any sports-related activity. This offshoot of orthopaedics treats a variety of ailments like tears in the rotator cuff, ligament injuries, and foot and ankle pain. Under this specialty, severe sports-related injuries, such as tears in the anterior cruciate ligament (ACL), posterior cruciate ligament (PCL), and medial collateral ligament (MCL), are treated.

Most of these ailments are caused by highly intense physical activity. The latter three issues commonly occur in athletes who play intense sports like football and basketball. Even hamstring ailments are treated in sports medicine.

It is understandable that sports medicine is often thought to involve only the treatment of star sportspersons. However, sports medicine also treats degenerative conditions like arthritis, back pain, joint pain, and soft tissue pains. There has been an increase in sports and its related activities in India. If one were to sketch a typical morning scene in India, the sidewalks and parks would be dotted with runners and fitness enthusiasts. Marathon runners have become a common sight, and people have been going to the gymnasiums more frequently.

As more people take up sports and other related activities, people are also more likely to face issues like shoulder, back, and neck pain. It has increased the need for sports orthopaedicians in our country. To become a sports orthopaedician, surgeons need additional training and experience. Sports orthopaedicians take care of elite athletes at the highest level. I have also been fortunate enough to meet a few of them. Sports medicine has also been greatly boosted by advances in technology.

For instance, if a person suffers from an ACL tear, it is no longer necessary to repair it via open surgery. A new branch of sports medicine called arthroscopy has made it easier. If you were to examine the literal meaning of the word, it means to look within the joint.

To treat an ACL tear, the orthopaedic surgeon will insert a camera attached to a thin tool. The surgeon will make a small 4-mm keyhole incision to insert the camera. The tool also consists of a lighting system and a lens, which is called the arthroscope. The doctor can then see a magnified image of the site with the help of the camera and decide on the treatment.

The ACL injury can be severe as the presence of a tear means that the ACL can never completely heal on its own. Most people will be able to lead a decent lifestyle without surgery.

However, if they want to lead even a semblance of an active physical life, which means being able to run and jog, they will need to undergo surgery to protect their knees from further ACL damage and potential arthritis. Surgery is seen as the last choice as there are various non-invasive methods available in sports medicine.

There is medication to treat pain, and in case of intense swelling and pain, they can opt for steroid injections into their knee joints. In case there is bleeding into the knee joint, the blood can be aspirated, which will help reduce the pain. A more common form of therapy could be the use of a knee brace.

The patient can also opt for physical therapy to strengthen the muscles around the knee joints. An ACL surgery, on the other hand, needs the surgeon to perform a reconstruction procedure. The surgeon will be able to remove the damaged ACL from the affected knee joint by the keyhole procedure. The ACL will then be replaced with a graft from the hamstring muscle.

Even if a patient opts to undergo an ACL surgery, he/she will still have to follow a long physical therapy program. Patients have to undergo rehabilitation therapy; they will need to get accustomed to using their legs and will have to learn to trust their knee joints. Generally, patients will be able to walk briskly by six weeks after the surgery.

They will be able to jog three months after the operation. Patients can resume active participation in contact sports after six months. Endoscopic procedures have risen to great prominence in orthopaedic surgery. Meniscal injuries and shoulder injuries were once treated via open surgeries. However, modern technology and medicine have ensured that these surgeries can now be performed via keyhole incisions. The idea is to do the same job and do it quickly. Keyhole surgery is also a safer and less painful way of treating such injuries. Technology is also playing a huge role in the training of young surgeons today.

In an earlier chapter, I mentioned the difficulties I had to undergo to be trained in laparoscopic or keyhole surgeries. It is especially tough when it comes to keyhole surgeries in sports medicine.

There are fewer surgical cases, and the surgeon is entrusted with the critical and difficult task of reconstruction. However, the use of Virtual Reality has made training in arthroscopy easier.

Arthroscopic simulators, such as the knee arthroscopy surgical trainer (KAST) developed by the AAOS and the Simbionix Arthromentor, are capable of providing haptic feedback of simulated cartilage and tendon and mimic surgical tools.[9] These are the new developments in surgery as a whole.

So, how do you choose a good orthopaedic surgeon? It is complicated! If you suffer from a fracture, any orthopaedician will be able to treat it. The problem of making an informed choice comes when you need to undergo a more complicated procedure. If you need a joint replacement or a joint reconstruction surgery, you need to look at a surgeon's track record.

Does the surgeon have experience in these procedures? Are there former patients who will vouch for the surgeon's skill and experience?

Broadly, we can divide the specialty of orthopaedic surgery into the following groups. I have also included a few pointers on choosing the right person for your problem.

Back pain: If it is the first time you are experiencing back pain, you may consult a general orthopaedic surgeon. However, subsequent episodes of back pain should be taken more seriously, and it is advisable to consult either an orthopaedic spine specialist or a neurosurgeon who has been treating these conditions regularly.

Joint replacement: A surgeon with many patients on his caseload or one with too few patients is not recommended. The former may not have enough time to communicate with you, and the latter may lack experience. A surgeon who has a moderate volume of patients is likely to have the time to communicate effectively and give you some attention and TLC. Such a surgeon would be the right choice. Ligament surgeries, arthroscopy etc, before undergoing these procedures, examine the surgeon's profile carefully and find out if you can connect with their former patients who underwent the same procedures successfully. Find out if these patients are now leading a normal pain-free life. A surgeon who operates on celebrities is definitely a safe bet, and you can be sure that this surgeon operates within their limits. Shoulder surgeon: Most surgeons are not experienced in the surgical management of shoulder conditions beyond the setting of a dislocated shoulder. In such cases, always get a second opinion from a renowned orthopaedic surgeon who is a specialist in treating shoulder conditions.

Hand surgeries: For procedures on the hand, it is advisable to consult a Hand surgeon or a Plastic surgeon who specialises in hand surgery.

# INCISIONS

| Values | Credits | Surgeon A | Surgeon B | Surgeon C | Surgeon D | Surgeon E |
|---|---|---|---|---|---|---|
| Education | 1-4 | | | | | |
| Experience | 1-3 | | | | | |
| Availability | 1-3 | | | | | |
| Behavior | 1-3 | | | | | |
| Personality | 1-2 | | | | | |
| Word of mouth | 1-4 | | | | | |
| Internet likes | 1-2 | | | | | |
| Ikigai | 1-3 | | | | | |
| Written Testimonials | 1-2 | | | | | |
| Video Testimonials | 1-4 | | | | | |
| Total | | | | | | |

# 11
# HARD NUTS!
## Neurosurgery

*"Only the neurosurgeon dares to improve upon five billion years of evolution in a few hours. The human brain. A trillion nerve cells storing electrical patterns more numerous than the water molecules of the world's oceans. The soul's tapestry lies woven in the brain's nerve threads. Delicate, inviolate, the brain floats serenely in a bone vault like the crown jewel of biology. What motivated the vast leap in intellectual horsepower between chimp and man? Between tree dweller and moon walker? Is the brain a gift from God, or simply the jackpot of a trillion rolls of DNA dice?"*

— Frank Vertosick Jr.

If cardiothoracic surgery is considered a glamorous specialty, then neurosurgery is truly awe-inspiring.

The common perception is that neurosurgeons are brain surgeons—they operate on the brain. Well, that would be an oversimplification of the role of neurosurgeons.

To better understand what the specialty of neurosurgery entails, let us take a look at the etymology of the word.

For instance, a cardiac surgeon is one who operates on the heart.

The word cardiac comes from the Greek word kardiā, which means heart. However, the root word for neurosurgeon comes from a Latin word, neuro, derived from the Greek word, neura, which means nerve.

So, neurology is the scientific study of the form and function of the nervous system. Thus, a neurosurgeon is involved with the various issues concerning the nervous system. The field of neurosurgery covers the broad spectrum of diseases and injuries that affect the brain, spinal cord, and peripheral nerves. It involves the diagnosis and treatment of various conditions that affect the central nervous system, peripheral nervous system, and autonomic nervous system. In short, a neurosurgeon will be handling the wiring of the body and a mistake can be costly.

**So how does one become a neurosurgeon?**

For this super-specialty, too, there are a couple of routes to reach the pinnacle. After completing the MBBS course, an aspiring applicant can directly write the entrance exams for the 6-year MCh Neurosurgery course (only available in a few centres).

Most surgeons go on to join the MCh Neurosurgery course after completing their Master's in General Surgery or Orthopaedics. The other recognised path to becoming a neurosurgeon would be to join the Diplomate of National Board (DNB) programme and pursue the neurosurgery course in recognised institutions in India. It is a super-specialty degree that is equivalent to the MCh degree.

Neurosurgery is a demanding specialty. A surgeon who takes up neurosurgery should be truly dedicated to his chosen specialty. The neurosurgeon is responsible for treating complex neurosurgical problems in patients.

It requires a lot of persistence, hard work, and long hours at the operating table. The neurosurgeon is required to have steady hands and immense stamina as neurosurgical procedures can extend for hours.

They should have the physical stamina to meet the demands of the specialty.

The psychomotor skills needed in this profession are honed by long hours of disciplined practice. They are exposed to a lot of stress, which they have to withstand, and after the procedure is completed, they have to deal with critically ill patients too.

Neurosurgery involves dealing with diseases affecting vital functions of the brain and spinal cord, such as the ability to think, speak, see, move, and feel. It involves operating on the most delicate organ of the body and requires a steady hand and nerves of steel.

When it comes to the surgical treatment of conditions affecting the brain or operations on the brain, there is no choice other than a neurosurgeon. It is a clear black and white choice. Let us look at some of the conditions that are treated by neurosurgeons.

The neurosurgeon has a distinct role to play in the treatment of conditions that affect the brain and the nervous system, such as stroke, brain tumours, epilepsy, and trauma. The spectrum of neurosurgical procedures involves removal of brain tumours, obliteration of an epilepsy focus, dealing with a bleed in the brain, and fixation of congenital anomalies of the brain and spine in children so as to restore the neurological function and eliminate pain and suffering.

The neurosurgeons spend more sleepless nights than the surgeons in any other surgical specialty. This is, of course, due to the high numbers of patients brought in with brain and spine trauma following road traffic accidents. The traffic moves day and night, and brain and spine trauma can occur at any time.

### Head injuries

Each day a huge number of people get injured on our roads, many of them grievously. Most of these are head injuries. Head injury is a serious ailment that can put a person in a coma for varying periods depending on the severity of the injury. Patients can sometimes be comatose and in a vegetative state for life.

Those who survive are often left with permanent physical,

emotional, and behavioural scars. What is more worrying is the fact that head injuries occur more commonly in men in the age group of 18 to 40 years, most often the breadwinners of their families. A neurosurgeon's workflow typically involves head injuries on a daily basis. Head injuries are treated in the ICU with medications and supportive measures.

In severe cases, brain surgery may be necessary. Here brain surgeons cut open the skull and enter the injured brain area. They may remove the injured part of the brain and stop the bleeding. The part of the skull that was removed for access is not replaced but preserved in the freezer for future use. Two or three months after the injury, a minor procedure is done to replace and fix the skull section back on the head. The treatment of a head injury begins in the intensive care unit and ends in the ward before the patient is discharged home.

## Spine surgery

Neurosurgeons are also spine (backbone) surgeons. In practice, much of a neurosurgeon's work involves performing spinal surgical procedures. Spine conditions, such as disc herniations, fractures, spinal stenosis, and tumours, and age-related back pain are very common in the population. In fact, back pain is one of the commonest reasons for a doctor's visit worldwide. The majority of back and neck pains in patients are treated by general practitioners in the community.

However, some patients with long-standing spinal issues may choose to consult the neurosurgeons directly. Although most of these patients can be managed without surgery in the outpatient clinics, some of them may be surgical candidates. Surgical options on the backbone depend on the spinal condition, location and severity of pain, and other factors, such as the patient's medical history and general health. Traditional spine surgery involved long, deep cuts through the muscles in the back or neck, which resulted in long scars and required an extended healing time. Often the results were unpredictable as well.

Presently, advancements in technology and surgical instrumentation have made it possible to perform some procedures in a less invasive manner. In minimally invasive spine surgery, a small incision is made, and a microscope or endoscope is used to access the area without dissecting a lot of muscle tissue.

This is called microscopic or endoscopic spine surgery. Another advancement in this field uses Image Guidance Technology to create a virtual image of the patient's spine as the surgery is being performed. By using this technology, the surgeon is able to operate with much more surgical precision and accuracy. These techniques have changed the landscape of spinal surgery.

## Cerebrovascular Accidents/Stroke

Stroke is a term that would be familiar to all. It is mainly considered a medical condition, and you would be familiar with neurologists treating stroke patients. What is the role of the neurosurgeons in this condition? To learn this, we must first understand how stroke occurs. A stroke can occur in a patient either due to ischaemia, that is, cessation of blood flow in one of the blood vessels in the brain, or due to a haemorrhage in any part of the brain.

When the stroke occurs due to a mechanical blockage of a cerebral artery by an embolus or thrombus, a procedure called Mechanical Embolectomy is performed. This is an image-guided procedure whereby a small tube is inserted into the concerned blood vessel in the brain through an artery in the leg. The block in the blood vessel is then flushed out.

This procedure can be performed up to 24 hours after a patient has had a stroke. However, the earlier it is performed, the better is the patient's recovery. We have already seen how neurosurgeons manage patients who have bleeding into the brain tissues. So, neurosurgeons have an important role in stroke patients in the immediate period. If a patient has a bleed or an aneurysm in the brain, it can only be treated by a neurosurgeon. Aneurysms in the brain (also known as cerebral aneurysms or intracranial aneurysms) are caused by a weakness in a blood vessel in the brain, resulting in a 'bubble' or 'bulge' that can rupture or bleed. When a brain aneurysm ruptures, there is bleeding into and around the brain tissue.

It often leads to subarachnoid haemorrhage, a severe form of injury to the brain, and can frequently result in severe disability or death. The two common treatments for this condition are microsurgical clipping and endovascular embolization, which are less invasive procedures than surgical clipping.

The overall health of the patient, his or her age, and the characteristics of the aneurysm all play a role in determining which treatment is used.

Microsurgical clipping entails a neurosurgeon removing a small section of the skull to create a window through which an aneurysm can be seen using an operating microscope. The neurosurgeon then identifies the blood vessel feeding the aneurysm and stops the blood flow by using a small metal clip on the neck of the aneurysm. Neurosurgeons use a 'mini-craniotomy' approach for the majority of aneurysm patients, which limits the length of the incision and the size of the skull opening. A smaller incision allows patients to go home after only two or three days in the hospital.

In rare cases, the neurosurgeon must clamp the entire artery leading to the aneurysm. In this case, a microsurgical bypass procedure to reroute blood to vital areas of the brain may be required. Endovascular embolization is a minimally invasive procedure performed inside blood vessels by interventional neuro-radiologists, neurologists, or neurosurgeons who have received special training.

A catheter, a small plastic tube, is inserted into an artery, usually in the groin. These guys then use X-rays (Digital subtraction angiography) to guide the catheter up into the neck arteries and into the arteries of the brain to visualise the procedure. Detachable coils are threaded through the catheter and inserted into the aneurysm to fill it, effectively reducing or stopping blood flow into the aneurysm. Stents (metal tubes), similar to those used by cardiologists, are sometimes used to open the blocked vessels. In some cases of severe stroke, the entire brain swells up and blood flow to the normal areas is hampered as well. This is an emergency situation. Neurosurgeons perform a procedure called Decompression Hemicraniectomy, where half of the patient's skull is removed to provide space for the swollen brain tissues.

The skull is frozen and preserved until the swelling comes down and it can be placed back.

In cases where there is bleeding into the brain, neurosurgeons can go with minimal intervention to evacuate the blood and save lives.

**Brain Tumours**

Tumours that occur in the brain are taken care of by the neurosurgeons. This is another area where their skills and abilities to fix the structures in the brain are tested. The surgical procedure used is called Craniotomy or open brain surgery. Tumours that occur in the brain may be classified as good tumours and bad tumours. You may be wondering how a tumour can be good!

In reality, any brain tumour is dangerous because it can spread to other areas of the brain or body or cause pressure effects on the surrounding brain structures. When neurosurgeons refer to good tumours, they are talking about benign tumours like meningiomas. These are most often non-cancerous and patients can have good survival rates following the surgical excision. And gliomas are the bad tumours. Gliomas are actually slow-growing malignant tumours. Both kinds of tumours require surgical excision to prevent their spread. Gliomas usually do not spread beyond the brain or spinal cord, but they can still be life-threatening because they can spread within the brain into areas where it is difficult to reach and tricky for the neurosurgeon to operate on.Whatever the kind of tumour, it is necessary that it should be excised. However, brain cancer surgery is tricky, and the procedure is difficult and requires a lot of preparation. Much depends on the location of the tumour, the skill of the operating surgeon, and the complete excision of the tumour.

If the tumour is situated in an easily accessible area of the brain, the surgeon will operate and remove as much of the tumour as possible. A small tumour can be easily separated from the surrounding brain tissue and excised completely.

However, bigger tumours or those that are located in sensitive areas of the brain pose a considerable risk if operated on.

Even in these situations, the neurosurgeon will strive to remove as much of the tumour as feasible without damaging the nearby vital structures.

Many times, the surgeon performs the surgery on an awake patient, especially when the tumour is close to the Eloquent Area of the brain (close to the area of the brain that controls speech, hand movements, memory, etc.), in order to avoid damage to this important region.

There is an element of uncertainty in the postoperative period when patients undergo craniotomy, where undesirable effects of surgery can lead to tremendous strain on the surgeon and his team.

Postsurgical patients could stay in the Neuro ICU for months and end in a vegetative state as the margin for error is too small for comfort.

**Epilepsy surgery**

Epilepsy or seizure disorders are usually managed with medications. However, the seizures may be refractory to medical therapy in a few patients. These patients would benefit from Epilepsy surgery.

The procedure involves removing or destroying the section of the brain from where the seizures originate, the focus of epilepsy. There are many types of surgical procedures that are used by neurosurgeons to treat refractory epilepsy. The commonest would be a resective surgery procedure and stereotactic surgery.

Resective surgery involves surgically excising a small portion of the brain from where the seizures are thought to originate.

It usually is in one of the temporal lobes of the brain. Alternatively, electrodes are placed in the affected part of the brain, and ablation is done to make that part non-functional.

## Treatment of Congenital Brain Anomalies

Children can be born with many congenital malformations in the brain. Surgical correction of these conditions is essential to correct the physical deformity and restore the maximum possible functionality to the affected child.

Sometimes, surgical correction can help in preventing neurological deficits. In this field, usually, paediatric neurosurgeons work alongside paediatric surgeons, paediatric plastic surgeons, and others.

Some of the conditions treated by neurosurgeons are Arnold Chiari malformations, encephaloceles, spinal deformities, and spinal map-formations.

In Chiari malformations, a portion of the brain will protrude through the bottom opening of the skull. This can place increased pressure on the brain or spinal cord.

There may be a blockage to the flow of the cerebrospinal fluid (CSF), the colourless liquid surrounding the brain and the spinal cord. This can result in a condition called hydrocephalus.

Neurosurgeons treat this condition by removing portions of the bone or soft tissue to relieve the excess pressure on the brain. This is called decompression surgery. They can also provide new pathways for the flow of the CSF.

An encephalocele is a type of neural tube defect where the brain is exposed outside and not covered by the skull. Neurosurgeons operate to remove bone and soft tissue and drain the collected CSF. The encephalocele is then surgically closed. To treat the hydrocephalus, a CSF shunt (tube) is placed in the ventricle of the brain, and through this, the CSF is drained into the child's abdomen or elsewhere. Arachnoid cysts are the most common type of brain cysts. The cysts are actually fluid-filled sacs and not tumours. These sacs occur at birth and are located in one of the three membranes that cover the brain. In rare cases, they can block the normal flow of CSF. Surgical treatment involves draining the cyst by making small openings and fashioning a natural fluid pathway.

## Pituitary Tumours

However, there are a few grey areas when it comes to neurosurgery. If a patient is to be operated on for a pituitary gland tumour, the neurosurgeon would usually pair up with an Otorhinolaryngologist. The pituitary gland can be found just above the nose, so it is natural for them to be buddies in this region. This operation requires a surgeon to operate through a telescope inserted through the nostrils.

A pituitary tumour is an abnormal growth of cells in the pituitary gland, the body's primary hormone-producing gland. The pituitary gland, about the size of a pea, is located in the centre of the brain, behind the nose and the eyes. Hormones are chemical substances produced by the body that control and regulate specific cells or organs. A pituitary tumour can disrupt the normal balance of hormones in the body, affecting a person's health. If these growths extend beyond the confines of the cavity, they can cause vision problems by pushing up on the optic nerves. Furthermore, tumours can impair pituitary gland function, resulting in a variety of hormonal dysfunctions involving the mechanisms listed above. Pituitary gland dysfunction is medically managed by an endocrinologist, whereas if you have a pituitary tumour that requires surgical excision, your neurosurgeon will work with an ENT specialist to remove the tumour. The ENT surgeon helps the neurosurgeon gain access to the pituitary tumour, so that it can be removed. Usually, the surgical approach in these cases is through the nose and the sinuses as the sella (where the pituitary gland lies in the comfort of the cradle-like bone within the skull) is close to the nose.

While this may appear to be a risky approach, it is actually a very safe and effective one. Endoscopic surgery is used to remove tumours from the pituitary gland and skull base through the nose. In this minimally invasive surgery, the surgeon uses a tiny endoscope with a camera and light to pass long instruments through the nostrils to excise the tumour. Pituitary tumours can cause hormonal imbalances as well as vision loss. Tumour removal frequently improves vision and restores normal hormone balance.

The term 'trans-sphenoidal' basically translates to 'through the sphenoid sinus.' It is a surgery that removes pituitary tumours through the nose and sphenoid sinus. The spine is another grey area. It is another domain where a neurosurgeon will be useful as the spinal cord is considered the secondary hub of the nervous system.

If a patient has lower back pain due to an unstable spine or a disc prolapse, or if they need a disc excision, they have a choice to go with either a well-trained Orthopaedic Surgeon or a Neurosurgeon.

## Deep Brain Stimulation

You would have come across numerous videos of brain surgery being performed on an awake patient who is either playing the guitar or some other instrument. The surgeon would usually be performing DBS on these patients.

Deep Brain Stimulation (DBS) is an area where neurosurgeons are increasingly playing a role. DBS involves placing electrodes in selected regions of the brain to stimulate them. In certain disease conditions, there are abnormal impulses released in the brain. These artificially produced impulses can help in regulating or decreasing the abnormal impulses. DBS is presently being used in the management of Parkinson's Disease, Refractory Epilepsy, Dystonia, etc.

Parkinson's Disease is a nervous system disorder with no cure. However, DBS has been found to relieve symptoms like stiffness and excessive shaking of the hands. Electrical impulses from DBS act to overrule the abnormal signals arising from the brain. For this reason, DBS is also referred to as the pacemaker for the brain.

The procedure involves placing a narrow electrode with specific localization into the brain with the help of computers, which is connected to a pulse generator. The pulse generator produces impulses at regular intervals. A well-trained neurosurgeon is needed to perform this procedure. Thus, you can see how a neurosurgeon is more than just a brain surgeon.   DBS is also being used in the management of refractive epilepsy. DBS releases regularly timed electrical signals that can act to disrupt the abnormal seizure-causing discharges from the brain.

This is usually an image-guided procedure undertaken by a trained neurologist. The generator that sends the impulses is usually embedded in the chest wall.

Minimally Invasive Neurosurgery

Neurosurgeons too have joined this bandwagon and are performing many procedures through minimally invasive surgery (MIS). These procedures involve the use of laparoscopic devices and robotic or remote-controlled devices.

There are many benefits to using the MIS technique in the field of neurosurgery. It allows the neurosurgeon to have a better view and increased magnification of the brain and the spinal cord. Considering the proximity of important structures in the brain, MIS can only help the neurosurgeon to be more accurate and effective in performing the procedure. This translates to a better outcome for the patient. In minimally invasive neurosurgery, endoscopes can provide detailed video images of the brain and its structures through very small incision.

Smaller instruments to cut, retrieve, or destroy abnormal tissues can be passed through the endoscope. There is almost no trauma to the surrounding structures. The incision is small and so is the postsurgical scar. Wound healing is quicker and the patient recovers faster with less pain.

Neurosurgery is one of the branches where the specialist surgeon dives into the super-specialty sometimes without even seeing the organ during his initial training as a doctor.

The aspiring neurosurgeon would not have had any exposure to the brain or surgery on the brain either during the undergraduate course (MBBS) or even during the General Surgery training. In your residency training, you never see a brain, let alone operate on one. A six-month rotation is insufficient to provide you with the experience you need to decide on your specialization in this subject. Nevertheless, the neurosurgeon is a tough guy with plenty of patience and attitude. The ability to sit for hours looking through a microscope and dissecting a yellow tumour from surrounding whitish-yellow normal brain tissue requires a lot of skill and is truly demanding. None of the other specialties give such unexpected results as those seen with neurosurgery.

Neurosurgeons are good at handling stress and making quick decisions. So basically, you would need a neurosurgeon when there is an emergency and when there is urgency. Most of the time, one does not really get to choose a neurosurgeon unless one is going in for a planned surgery for a tumour.

Trauma is one emergency where urgent surgical treatment can well save a patient's life. A vascular bleed in the brain is another situation similar to trauma to the brain. Here the blood that oozes out can lead to compression of the normal brain tissue. The bleeds can occur inside the brain or outside and so they may compress the brain from within or from outside. Vascular bleeds in the brain can occur due to trauma or uncontrolled hypertension apart from aneurysmal bleeds. Whatever the cause, it requires urgent evacuation to prevent brain swelling and death.

Neurosurgeons, in general, may appear to be impatient and on the move at all times. This is because of the highly stressful conditions under which they operate.

| Values | Credits | Surgeon A | Surgeon B | Surgeon C | Surgeon D | Surgeon E |
|---|---|---|---|---|---|---|
| Education | 1-4 | | | | | |
| Experience | 1-3 | | | | | |
| Availability | 1-3 | | | | | |
| Behavior | 1-3 | | | | | |
| Personality | 1-2 | | | | | |
| Word of mouth | 1-4 | | | | | |
| Internet likes | 1-2 | | | | | |
| Ikigai | 1-3 | | | | | |
| Written Testimonials | 1-2 | | | | | |
| Video Testimonials | 1-4 | | | | | |
| Total | | | | | | |

# 12
## THIS CRAB IS SERIOUS BUSINESS
### Surgical Oncology

*"Cancer did not bring to me my knees, it brought me to my feet."* – Michael Douglas

Cancer surgery sounds self-explanatory! By itself, it appears very easy to define. If you have cancer, go see a cancer surgeon! However, it is not that simple. Perhaps it is best if we take some time to understand the care process of cancer at first. Oncology is the study of cancer and you will see that many hospitals will have an Oncology Department. The doctors and specialists who treat cancer are called oncologists.

Oncology is a super-speciality degree and doctors obtain this degree after completing their post-graduation in General Medicine or General Surgery. An oncologist can have a DM degree in Oncology or an MCh degree in Surgical Oncology. You also have doctors specialising in Radiation Oncology or Radiotherapy and holding an MD degree in the same. Pathologists too can specialise in the field of cancer and hold a DM degree in Onco-Pathology.

Now, you can see that the onco-surgeons are the ones who specialise in surgical oncology and it is to them one would go for cancer surgeries. But not always!

Before talking about cancer surgeries, I want to give you some basic information about cancer. It is a frightful topic, to be sure. But it is important that people have some basic information about cancer, its diagnosis, the treatment options, etc. Given the increasing incidence of cancer in the present times, it seems inevitable that everyone has at least one family member or acquaintance affected by cancer.

Cancer is a process where the tissue cells begin to grow and multiply uncontrollably. Every cell has a life cycle in which it is born, gives birth to other cells like itself /multiplies, and then self-destructs. This process is known as 'Apoptosis.' When such a system fails, there is no destruction and the production capacity remains the same, and the number of cells in the organ increases and produces a mass. This mass is termed 'tumour.' Cancers can affect any part of our body. They can affect the skin, muscles, and bones, the different organs in our body, the sensory organs, the brain, the blood vessels, etc. Cancers are named according to the type of cells or tissues involved. For instance, squamous cell carcinoma affects the skin or the lining of different hollow organs in our bodies. Tumours affecting the muscles are called sarcomas, and those affecting glandular tissues are usually adenocarcinomas.

Some cancers grow slowly and are restricted to the area of origin. They do not spread elsewhere in the body. These are known as benign tumours. Cancers that grow exponentially and spread to adjoining tissues as well as to the rest of the body are termed malignant tumours. Malignant cancers can be life-threatening in advanced stages if untreated. Benign tumours usually do not have any life-threatening consequences. But they can have deleterious consequences caused by the pressure effects of a growing tumour. They might also have a negative cosmetic effect.

## Diagnosis of Cancer:

Cancer can present with many signs and symptoms specific to the organ affected. For instance, breast cancer may present with a swelling or lump in the breast region. Sometimes, the signs and symptoms are not so specific. A person might just experience weight loss, loss of appetite, chronic tiredness, headaches, fever, etc. Any unexplained symptom should be investigated. Blood cancers can actually present with just tiredness. Certain symptoms may not present in the affected organ per se, and the patient may present with symptoms caused by the spread of the tumour to the other organs. For example, patients suffering from prostate cancer can present with severe bone pain or fractures due to bone metastasis or with secondaries in the lungs.

The diagnosis of cancer can be confirmed with some tests and investigations. Sometimes there is an obvious deformity or swelling.

In some cancers, such as blood cancers, blood tests can help make the diagnosis. Imaging modalities, such as X-ray, CT scans, mammography, ultrasound scans, and MRI, play a crucial role in cancer diagnosis as well. In many instances, a biopsy is what helps confirm the diagnosis of cancer.

A biopsy is a procedure where a sample of tissue is removed from the body and sent to the pathologist for examination under the microscope. After examining the sample, the pathologist can give an opinion on what kind of cancer it is, and sometimes the grade of the disease as well.

Grading of cancer basically is describing the extent of abnormality in the cells. The cells in low-grade cancers grow slowly and they resemble normal cells to a great extent. High-grade cancers will have cells that show a lot of abnormalities and they will grow faster as well.

There are different ways of performing a biopsy. Needle aspiration and cytology is the commonest procedure. A fine needle is inserted into the tissue in question and some material is aspirated. This is then sent to the pathology laboratory.

This procedure is useful when the tumour is accessible or visible from the outside, such as a breast lump. Another option is image-guided biopsy where CT imaging or ultrasonography is used to direct the needle into the lesion. Surgical biopsies involve open surgery or a laparoscopic procedure to obtain the sample tissue for examination.

## Who performs the biopsies?

Often the concerned surgeon to whom the patient went for consultation may perform the biopsy. Biopsies may be performed by pathologists as well and they also perform image-guided biopsies. However, the samples are always examined and reported on by a trained pathologist.

### Treatment Modalities:

Once the diagnosis of cancer is confirmed, the treatment is begun. There are various methods by which cancers are treated. Usually, to reach complete remission, that is, complete removal of all the cancer cells in the body, the patient is offered multiple modalities simultaneously or in quick succession.

The following are the ways in which any cancer may be treated:
- Surgical removal of the tumour
- Medical therapy
- Radiation therapy
- Combination of all or two of the above methods

Medical oncologists use, as the name suggests, medicines to treat cancer. Some of the popular forms of medical oncology include chemotherapy, targeted therapy, and immunotherapy. Chemotherapy is a treatment that uses drugs that contain powerful chemicals to kill cancerous cells in the body. Targeted therapy involves using drugs that target specific markers present on the cancer cells. Immunotherapy involves using drugs to stimulate the body's immune system to fight cancer.

Radiation oncologists use radiation therapy to treat cancer. This form of therapy involves the usage of high-energy X-rays to kill the cancerous cells in the body. Surgical oncologists treat cancer by removing the cancerous tumour through surgery. The training for surgical oncology is largely organ-specific.

There are some areas in the body where cancers are treated not by the onco-surgeons, but by the concerned specialists. For example, most of the cancers in the brain are usually operated on by neurosurgeons. Therefore, for surgical excision of a brain tumour, you would have to go to a neurosurgeon rather than to an onco-surgeon. The urinary system is another area where the specialists, that is the urologists, are quite competent and usually perform cancer surgeries. That means a person having cancer of the kidney or the urinary bladder will more likely be treated by a urologist. Cardiovascular surgery is another department where they take care of cancer surgeries in the chest region as well. Cardiovascular surgeons are quite competent to perform cancer surgeries in the chest, and most surgical oncologists do not perform these surgeries.

This brings us to the fundamental question: what then exactly is the role of the cancer surgeons? What surgeries do they perform? There are a lot of surgeries performed by cancer surgeons.

They specialise in taking care of cancers of the head and neck. Thus, they treat cancers of the mouth, tongue, and oesophagus, and also cancers in other organs like the breast. They also are competent to perform abdominal cancer surgeries. However, they face intense competition in this area from the gastrointestinal (GI) surgeons, who are also trained to perform these cancer surgeries.

In fact, the GI surgeon who is also trained in oncological surgery can actually competently perform even the more challenging surgeries, such as surgeries for retroperitoneal tumours, intestinal tumours, and liver tumours. It is at this point that we also look at the different types of surgical methods adopted by surgeons to treat cancers. The first type is open surgery. It involves cutting open a site to excise the tumour. In this process, the surgeon may have to also resect and remove some nearby healthy tissue and lymph nodes.

The second type of surgery is minimally invasive surgery. Small incisions are made to insert a long narrow tube with a camera attached to the end of it. The camera will project a magnified image to the surgeon on a high-definition screen. The surgeon will then insert special surgical tools, which will be inserted simultaneously through other minor incisions made. These tools will enable the surgeon to excise the tumour. This method is also known as the laparoscopic surgical method.

There are other forms of minimally invasive surgical methods as well. One of them is cryosurgery. It is a targeted method where specific cancerous cells can be destroyed. The method involves the use of liquid nitrogen or argon gas. These two substances can produce extreme cold and that cold is used to kill the cancerous cells. It is used in the treatment of retinoblastoma, skin cancers, liver cancer that is confined to the liver, non-small cell lung cancer, early-stage prostate cancer, and chondrosarcomas. When it comes to skin tumours, the surgeon can apply the liquid nitrogen to the concerned area with the help of a spray device or a cotton swab.

If the cancer is within the body, the surgeon will have to make a small incision. Through this incision, the surgeon will insert a tool called the cryoprobe. The surgeon will then let the argon gas or liquid nitrogen flow through the cryoprobe and apply it to the tumour. Unlike in laparoscopy, here the surgeon will have to use ultrasonography and MRI to guide the cryoprobe to the correct site without harming the healthy tissues adjacent to the tumour.

It is also possible to insert more than one cryoprobe to treat cancers in different parts of the body. However, these modalities have a very limited role in the treatment of cancers.

Laser therapy is another method used to treat cancer. It, too, is a targeted method of treatment. It uses a narrow beam of light that is intense enough to kill cancerous cells and potentially malignant cells. The therapy is based on the idea that tumours absorb a different wavelength of light when compared to the healthy cells in the body. Thus, surgeons can use the laser to target specific tumorous growths and destroy them.

It is used to treat cancers that occur on the body's surface, such as basal cell skin cancer, or cancers involving the cells that line the inner organs, such as colorectal polyps and non-small cell lung cancer. It is also used to treat precancers in the areas of the anus, penis, vagina, vulva, and cervix. There are three types of lasers used in this method. The first is the carbon dioxide laser and the second is the argon laser. These two lasers are used on the surface as they can dissect the skin without going into the deeper layers. They are generally used to treat skin cancers. The final type of laser used is the neodymium:yttrium-aluminum-garnet (Nd:YAG) laser.

This laser is used to treat inner organs like the uterus, oesophagus, and colon. This laser is guided toward the cancerous cells through an endoscope. This endoscope uses thin optical fibres to transmit light onto the malignant cells. These light fibres are used as a single fibre or in a bundle.

The endoscope is inserted into the body through the natural openings in the body like the mouth, nose, anus, and vagina. Laser therapy is also used in conjunction with normal surgery.

The laser is used to seal nerve endings after the excision of a tumour to lessen pain. It can also be used to seal the lymph vessels after excision to limit the growth and spread of cancer cells and reduce swelling. Lasers can also be used during surgery to seal the blood vessels to reduce bleeding.[10]

These are some of the minimally invasive surgeries available today. Now, this is the pertinent question: Are cancer surgeons trained in these methods? As mentioned earlier, cancer surgeons specialise in surgeries in the head and neck region. There are also cancer surgeons who have specialised in breast cancer surgery. Some cancer surgeons can also do a wonderful job when it comes to gynaecological cancer surgery. Some onco-surgeons are also well-equipped and trained to conduct cancer surgeries in the abdominal area.

However, cancer surgeries in the abdominal area are now frequently done via minimally invasive surgery methods.

Well, you will likely come across a few cancer surgeons who will also have adequate training in these types of minimally invasive procedures.

If you can find someone like that, they are your best bet for an onco-surgical procedure in the abdomen. However, there are very few of these onco-surgeons with the requisite training and experience to perform minimally invasive procedures for cancer in the abdomen. The numbers are few, and you might not be easily able to consult such a person. But the training methods have changed over the years and the newer trained onco-surgeons in premier institutes like the Tata memorial hospital are well equipped in taking up minimal access surgeries on their own.

So, this will inevitably make you ask the question, "Is the surgical method important?" How does a minimally-invasive surgery differ from an open surgery when it comes to surgical oncology? Is there a difference in their clinical outcomes? If you opt for undergoing surgery using the minimally invasive procedure or a robotic procedure, you will have the benefit of experiencing less pain. The recovery after surgery is also faster with minimally-invasive procedures. However, there is no great difference demonstrated in the clinical outcomes. One must also keep in mind that the outcome following a surgical procedure is also determined by the skill and the experience of the surgeon. Hence, the organ-specific surgeon trained and experienced in minimally invasive surgical methods becomes a better choice than a cancer surgeon in such cases. I am of the firm opinion that patients should be more focused on the results than the method. The primary concern is to be cured of cancer. The malady is more important than the method. To be free of cancer should be the focus and not the procedures that are followed. Do not let yourself be bogged down with unnecessary details and the choice of the surgical method. Rather, invest your time toward making an informed decision in finding the right surgeon.

Find the best surgeon who can rid you of your cancer. It does not matter an iota if the surgeon has to do it via open surgery, minimally invasive surgery, or robotic surgery.

Obviously, when it comes to oncological surgeries in the head and neck region, the surgical oncologist stands tall. They do a wonderful and competent job in handling cancers of the tongue, throat, or thyroid gland. The same holds true when it comes to breast cancer as well.

Onco-surgeons experienced in breast cancer surgeries are a good choice. In fact, most breast cancer surgeries also include a procedure called axillary lymph node clearance. Basically, all the lymph nodes in the axilla on the same side as the breast cancer are removed. This is a diagnostic as well as a therapeutic procedure. This is important because pathological examination allows us to identify any spread of cancer to these nodes.

Removal of the nodes in their entirety ensures that there is less chance of future spread of cancer to the other regions of the body. Cancer surgeons are trained to perform lymph node dissections competently. However, as mentioned before, they do face intense competition from the GI surgeons when it comes to cancer surgeries at other locations, such as the abdomen or the pelvis. The GI surgeons are not only well-versed in minimally invasive surgeries, but they are also very familiar with the anatomy of the area.

They know the ins and outs of the area as they are the surgeons who carry out operations in the abdominal area for non-cancer-related issues. Thus, they are well-versed in working through tiny incisions in the abdomen. They are already quite experienced and competent in performing various surgical procedures in this field through the tiny incision. So, they are proficient when it comes to cancer surgeries in the abdominal area even if they do not have the title of being a cancer surgeon. If you have to choose a surgeon for cancer in the abdominal area, a GI surgeon with experience in performing minimally invasive and robotic surgeries will be a better choice over a surgical oncologist who also performs head and neck surgery, thyroid surgery, and breast surgery.

Why do I say so? It can be compared to choosing the Master of one trade over a Jack of all trades. Just ask yourself the question: Would you like to take a chance with a cancer surgeon who is a Jack of all trades? Or would you like a surgeon who is able to give you a good surgical outcome with little pain and scarring? The diagnosis of cancer is a mentally traumatic event for both the patient and the family. Most of them would want to get the best possible treatment. A few may be worried about the cost and if the patient would be able to tolerate the treatment. In the following section, we will try and offer some clarity as to what the thought process of the patient and the relatives should be when they seek cancer treatment.

### Who is the first specialist you should approach for cancer?

There is no straightforward answer to this. It depends on the type of cancer and the facilities available in the hospital. Meeting the right doctor early reduces the evaluation time and lessens any chances of errors. You could see any one of the below specialists and as they work closely together, you would be treated accordingly and referred to the right person.

Surgical Oncologists—who specialize in cancer surgery
Medical Oncologists—who specialize in chemotherapy
Radiation oncologists—who specialize in radiation treatment

Depending on their sub-specialisation, there may be breast, gynaecologic, head and neck, uro oncology, gastrointestinal, and bone and soft tissue surgical oncologists. What patients need to understand is that there may be more than one doctor and more than one department in the hospital with equal competency in handling cancer cases. This begs the question as to how one should choose their doctor. We will discuss that a little while later. For blood cancers and lymphomas, the main treatment will be chemotherapy and it is best that patients with these conditions consult a medical oncologist or haematologist.

The initial evaluation for solid organ cancers like breast cancer and head and neck cancers is usually done by doctors with a surgical background in most centres. There are a couple of reasons for this:

Very often benign conditions overlap with cancerous conditions. This is especially true for cancer of the breast, thyroid, etc. Benign tumours are often dealt with by surgeons.

Performing a biopsy is usually done best by surgeons.

A centre where surgical, medical, and radiation facilities are available under one roof is called "Comprehensive Cancer Centre".

In these centres, there is better coordination in treatment between the three specialities, leading to better results.

## Who would be the best doctor to treat my cancer?

As mentioned earlier, there is likely to be more than one competent doctor to handle a particular type of cancer.

Titles can be misleading and may not reflect the true competence of the doctor. Reviews and ratings on google are not a good way to decide as these can be easily falsified. Many senior and experienced doctors do not bother to seek ratification from their patients. There are instances in which honest doctors who advise the right treatment for the patients get bad reviews because it does not match the unrealistic expectation of the relatives.

The following points may help you decide if your treating doctor is honest and experienced in handling cancer cases:

A good cancer specialist explains the diagnosis of cancer in detail. There may be instances in which the diagnosis is uncertain and yet we may have to proceed with the treatment. This is true of cancers in the breast, thyroid, and ovary where it is not uncommon to get lumps that are borderline and the diagnosis can be made only during or after surgery. If the diagnosis is not clear-cut, there is no harm in explaining so to the patient.

Staging is an important part of cancer treatment and in most instances, it would be wrong to jump into treatment without proper staging.

There are a few exceptions to this. Staging involves doing appropriate investigations, such as a PET CT scan, MRI, or regular CT scan.

Always trust a doctor who gives the overall plan of treatment rather than the plan pertaining to his speciality. For instance, for a patient diagnosed with early breast cancer, a good practice would be to tell the patient that following the surgery she is likely to need chemotherapy and radiation depending on the pathology report rather than just explaining about the surgery. This will keep the patient mentally prepared and also help plan the finances.

Cancer is a multimodality treatment. This means that the patient quite often needs a combination of treatments. There are many cancers that were traditionally treated by surgery, but now trials have shown benefit in giving chemotherapy and/or radiation before surgery. This is true for stage 3 cancer of the rectum or breast.

Despite these changes in the treatment protocols, many surgeons push for surgery without considering pre-surgery or neoadjuvant chemotherapy and radiation. A good doctor would always consider these options in the interest of the patient, and if it is not indicated, will explain why he thinks so.

A good doctor would explain all the options of treatment. In certain cancers, surgery and radiation may have equal chances of cure. It would be best to put all the options on the table and then help the patient decide what is best for them.

In certain cases, like in very old people and very advanced cancers, not doing anything may be the best option. Minimally invasive surgery has come up in a big way for cancers of the abdomen and thorax. About two decades ago, it was considered that doing cancer surgery by laparoscopy was harmful. Robotic surgery too has come up in a big way in the past few years.

The decision of whether a particular surgery is suitable for the laparoscopic or robotic method has to be individualised. It would be wrong to not offer the patient minimally invasive surgery when it is suitable. Equally wrong would be to perform laparoscopic or robotic surgery in a patient who is not suitable to undergo this.

A good surgeon would discuss these options with the patient and explain to them if he thinks that a particular surgery is suitable to be performed via the minimally invasive method. If he feels that the patient or the tumour is not suitable for a minimally invasive procedure, he would explain this too.

A few surgeons do not explain the chances of surgical complications and chances of recurrence fearing that patients will refuse treatment. This has been a frequent cause of litigation.

A good surgeon will have his way of explaining this to the patient without offending him or turning him away. Always believe a surgeon who says that complications are possible rather than one who says he has never had any complications.

A good doctor would encourage a second opinion and not be offended by it. If you desire to take a second opinion, then please be frank with the doctor about it. If the second opinion is greatly different from the first opinion, you can go back to the first doctor and ask him for clarity.

Certain surgeries may require surgeons from two different areas of expertise. A good surgeon would not hesitate in asking for help from another if it adds value. If your surgeon says that he will need the help of another surgeon do not take it as a sign of incompetence; rather, you should appreciate the surgeon for being honest about it. If your treating cancer specialist has done all or most of the above things, then you can be assured that you are in safe hands. Please remember that in certain situations in cancer there may not be clear-cut answers. A certain doctor may suggest surgery while another may consider it inoperable, and yet both may be right in their own ways.

What is important is the justification provided by the surgeon and how well you are convinced by it.

### Where should you take cancer treatment?

Comprehensive cancer centres are best suited to treat as there would be better coordination between different specialities.

This does not mean that cancer surgery should never be done outside these centres. If cancer surgery is done outside comprehensive cancer centres, we still have to make sure that a proper discussion regarding all options of treatment has been done.

As cancer surgeries tend to be complex it will be of great help if there is a good intensive care unit. As most cancer patients tend to be elderly, it would be of help to have competent cardiology, nephrology, and pulmonology departments.

Pathology reporting plays a vital role and an experienced onco-pathologist is a must for proper results. The bottom line is that rather than just going by name or qualifications or advertisement, please check if your treating surgeon ticks the right boxes for the above-mentioned points. If he does so, then you can trust him/her to give the best possible results for your near and dear ones suffering from cancer.

To summarize, cancer surgeons do not operate on cancers of the brain, the kidneys, and the structures and bones that are present in the thoracic cavity. But they are experienced in performing cancer surgeries in all other areas and would be a good choice for operating on other cancers. For oncological surgeries in the head and neck region, the thyroid gland, and the breasts, the cancer surgeon is the best choice and they are the best in the field. They are the optimum choice if the oncological surgery is done via the open surgery method. Open surgery is the preferred method in cases where the size of the tumour to be resected is large and it is not feasible to undertake the procedure through a minimally invasive method. However, when it comes to oncological surgeries in the abdomen involving the large intestine, the small intestine, or the biliary system, or in some cases, the pancreas, a GI surgeon who is also trained in minimally invasive surgery would be equally competent to do a fair job. When it comes to cases like these, the experience of the surgeon should be the guiding point and the focus, whatever be the area of surgery or the surgical method he/she adopts. Do not let the surgical method of choice of the surgeon serve as a roadblock for choosing a surgeon when it comes to treating your cancer.

| Values | Credits | Surgeon A | Surgeon B | Surgeon C | Surgeon D | Surgeon E |
|---|---|---|---|---|---|---|
| Education | 1-4 | | | | | |
| Experience | 1-3 | | | | | |
| Availability | 1-3 | | | | | |
| Behavior | 1-3 | | | | | |
| Personality | 1-2 | | | | | |
| Word of mouth | 1-4 | | | | | |
| Internet likes | 1-2 | | | | | |
| Ikigai | 1-3 | | | | | |
| Written Testimonials | 1-2 | | | | | |
| Video Testimonials | 1-4 | | | | | |
| Total | | | | | | |

# 13
## NOT FAKE AT ALL!
### Plastic Surgery

*"How you start is important, very important, but in the end, it is how you finish that counts. It is easier to be a self-starter than a self-finisher. The victor in the race is not the one who dashes off swiftest but the one who leads at the finish. In the race for success, speed is less important than stamina. The sticker outlasts the sprinter in life's race. In America we breed many hares but not so many tortoises."*
- B. C. Forbes

On March 20, 2010, the world woke up to the news of the first full face transplant ever to be performed. In Barcelona, 30 Spanish doctors led by Dr. Joan-Pere Barret, carried out the surgery on a man injured in a shooting accident. Dr. Barret, a plastic surgeon, was also the lead surgeon. The specialty of plastic and cosmetic surgery is usually synonymous with cosmetic and reconstructive surgery. The terms plastic surgery and cosmetic surgery are often used interchangeably. When we hear of this specialty, procedures such as breast lifts, abdominal tucks, facelifts, and re-implantation of limbs come to our mind immediately. But, in reality, cosmetic surgeons do a lot more than that, like Michael Bevan of the Australian cricket team, who is a finisher.

The plastic surgeons are the 'Michael Bevans' of the medical world. At the end of the match, Bevan, who goes in to bat at number seven, finishes the job started by the batsmen before him. This is exactly what plastic surgeons are often called to do.

Plastic surgeons specialise in reconstructive surgery. Patients with deformities caused by congenital diseases, injuries, infections, or burns are treated by them. Many plastic surgeons opt to specialise in cosmetic surgery, which involves performing operations for improving a patient's looks or aesthetic appearance or doing microvascular procedures. They also perform reconstructive procedures following cancer surgeries (free flaps) or burn injuries. Plastic surgery is one of the most sought-after medical specialties. It is possible that the training will take more than a decade. Aspiring plastic surgeons should first obtain a Masters's degree in General Surgery and then complete MCh. in Plastic Surgery.

The term 'plastic' in the context of plastic surgery is sometimes misunderstood to mean 'artificial.' The word is derived from the ancient Greek word plastikos, which means to mold. This is a medical specialty that focuses on enhancing a person's looks as well as reconstructing face and body tissue deformities caused by sickness, accident, or congenital anomalies.

Plastic surgery improves and restores both function and aesthetics. It can include surgery on any region of the anatomy except the central nervous system. Plastic surgeons perform procedures involving the skin, scar tissues, burns, birthmarks, and tattoo removal. They treat maxillofacial (facial skeleton) and congenital abnormalities, such as malformed ears, cleft palate, and cleft lip. Reconstructive surgery aims to restore function and appearance, as well as rectify anomalies caused by birth defects, trauma, or medical illnesses such as cancer. A cancer surgeon would remove the organ, but they would have no idea how to cover the deficiency. As a result, they usually approach the plastic surgeons to find some tissue, bone, muscles, or skin to cover it.

They transport tissue across the body and re-create bodily components that have been altered due to sickness or therapy.

This is common in malignancies of the head and neck, for example. Reconstructive surgeons are frequently involved in surgical instances involving patients when their function is not immediately apparent.

Plastic surgeons are adept at stretching skin and closing wounds, and they frequently are a part of the surgical team treating a cancer patient. After the primary surgeon removes the tumour, a reconstructive surgeon will repair the incision using sophisticated procedures and then monitor the patient's recovery to ensure that they are recovering appropriately. Some of the procedures that plastic surgeons are well qualified to undertake are breast and face reconstruction, skin, tendon, and bone grafting, scar revisions, and even treating and repairing regions damaged by radiation and chemotherapy.

Plastic surgeons, like those from the other key specialties engaged in trauma treatment, play an important role in a trauma centre, especially in India. Many times, the plastic surgeon's efforts save limbs and even save lives, and post-traumatic sequelae are either prevented or addressed. Lacerations, severe abrasions, and rips of the skin and fat layers are all examples of sharp and blunt trauma. There may be deeper soft tissue injuries to the muscles, tendons, blood vessels, and nerves. While these exterior injuries are readily apparent, the seriousness of the damage is not necessarily so. Reconstructive surgery and selecting the optimal approach should be considered early in the cancer treatment planning process and not as an afterthought. Surgery, radiation, and chemotherapy are complementary kinds of treatment, and the sequencing, timing, and length of each can be influenced by reconstructive surgery possibilities.

Some tumours are untreatable unless reconstructive surgery is part of the treatment strategy. Reconstruction is frequently not a 'one-and-done' operation, but rather a series of treatments carried out in stages—either at the outset of therapy or later—to achieve the best possible results.

Microvascular surgery, also known as microvascular reconstructive surgery, is the repair of significant surgical defects utilizing surgical grafts made of muscle, bone, skin, or fat, as well as blood vessel suturing to aid in the healing of the surgical site. Microvascular surgery is a relatively recent procedure that is used to repair large surgical abnormalities. Patients who have had substantial tissue trauma as a result of the above-mentioned causes or illnesses, and whose surgical defect is large enough to need a surgical transplant, may consider microvascular surgery. Microvascular surgery can be performed to relocate and reattach amputated body parts. Such as fingers, hands, and arms that have been severed or disconnected. This is accomplished by reconnecting and uniting the minute blood vessels, so that circulation is restored to the wounded tissue before it dies or necroses.

Some of the best plastic surgeons I have known do a fantastic job of sitting up all night attempting to restore an arm to the working state or restore a decent appearance to a patient. We frequently see plastic surgeons perform microvascular surgeries to attach an arm or a finger or to attach, reattach, or retain a leg.

Many nerves and veins are involved, and this is never undertaken by anyone else; it is only done by plastic surgeons who spend hours upon hours looking under a microscope, trying to fix things.

The scope of plastic and reconstructive surgery is enormous! These surgeons are able to reconstruct the tendon and nerve injuries and get conditions of the carpal tunnel sorted out (Hand Surgeons), while they also can reconstruct the face after an accident or rectify a cleft lip and palate in a newborn child (Maxillofacial Surgeons). They also look after the burn patients right from the start till the patient walks out of the hospital, that is, from dressing the burns to the final release of the contractures and reconstruction procedures (Burn Specialists). The role of cosmetic surgery is to boost a person's self-esteem and confidence by improving their appearance. Any portion of the face or body can be treated with cosmetic surgery. The main aims of cosmetic procedures are to improve visual appeal, symmetry, and proportion.

The scope of their work would include treatment of gynaecomastia in males to liposuction, tummy tuck, and nose reconstruction in either sex to mummy makeover in females.

Aesthetic surgery can be performed on any part of the body, including the head, neck, and face. Cosmetic surgery is classified as elective since it treats regions that function normally. However, in cancer surgeries, especially if a huge tumour is involved and coverage is required, most often, the plastic surgeons have a role.

So, you have the cancer surgeon who will remove the tumour and the plastic surgeon who will give you a cover that looks respectable enough, allowing you to live a long and healthy life, albeit not as it was in the original, but with a very good resemblance to how you were before, and it would take a lot of effort to do so.

Plastic surgeons also are part of the Bariatric surgery team, which specialises in weight loss surgery. Following bariatric surgery, a patient's weight approaches the ideal weight after 18 months. This is when the patient's weight gets steady and is as near to the ideal weight as feasible; this is the right time to think about plastic surgery. Before having surgery, doctors encourage patients to be at a steady weight for three months. This is due to a variety of factors. First, rapid weight reduction puts your body in a poor nutritional balance, making it less capable of repairing fresh surgical wounds. Second, when one's body mass index (BMI) drops, the chance of surgical complications diminishes. Third, as you move closer to your ideal weight, the cosmetic outcomes of the surgery (how things look) tend to improve. You could have a variety of procedures like tummy tuck, facelift, and arms lift after the weight loss is complete. The apron of skin that falls on the abdomen after the weight loss can be really unsightly.

**Procedures in Cosmetic Surgery:**

Breast Augmentation, Breast Lift, and Breast Reduction are all procedures that may be used to improve the appearance of the breasts.

Rhinoplasty and Chin or Cheek Enhancement are examples of facial contouring procedures.

Facelift, Eyelid Lift, Neck Lift, and Brow Lift are examples of facial rejuvenation procedures.

Tummy Tuck, Liposuction, and Gynaecomastia Treatment are options for body contouring.

Laser resurfacing and Botox and Filler Treatments are options for skin rejuvenation.

However, cosmetic surgery can be considered a luxury. Many people may live with minor malformations such as a slightly twisted nose or a mouth that is slightly unusual. Or they may have a bump here and there or a scar that irritates them all the time. These are the problems with which you can live. However, some patients may not want to live with these minor problems and wish to get rid of them. This is where the role of plastic surgeons comes into play. Regrettably, many individuals who opt for cosmetic surgery have the expectation that they will look 20 years younger following the procedure. This is unlikely to happen, and many of them are left dissatisfied.

If you ever opt to undergo a plastic surgery procedure, you must have extremely realistic expectations. The deformity may be a minor one, but the idea should be for you to have an acceptable result rather than results that are out of this world.

Often I see the results in Bollywood or Hollywood heroines who have had cosmetic surgeries. The scars may not be plainly visible, but they are always there if you look closely enough. As a result, you must come to terms with the fact that you either have a scar or a bump.

According to 'The 10 Faces Of Michael Jackson', a documentary released in 2015, the late singer had over 100 surgeries performed on his face. When Michael Jackson died in 2009, many concerns regarding the eccentric music star's purported plastic surgery remained unanswered. His remarkable makeover made him renowned throughout his career, with people wondering how much surgery he had undergone and why his skin had become white.

In 1979, Michael had his first nose job. He said he had the procedure because he injured his nose during a dance rehearsal and needed an operation. However, Michael was dissatisfied with his initial nose operation and had it redone to rectify it. Michael's chin unexpectedly acquired a fissure in 1988. He went in for treatments every two months, according to Dr. Wallace Goodstein, who worked alongside Michael's physician in the 1990s.

"While I was there, I performed roughly 10 to 12 procedures in two years," he revealed in 2009. Michael's nose became substantially smaller and his complexion whiter over the 1990s. Michael admitted to Oprah Winfrey at one time that his lighter complexion was caused by the skin ailment vitiligo. He also confided to his buddy, illusionist Uri Geller, that he was changing his looks to 'not look like his father.' By this time, his face had changed so drastically that it was difficult to tell which surgeries he had undergone; nonetheless, according to Dr. Goodstein, "he had many nose jobs, cheek implants, and a cleft inserted in his chin. He underwent eyelid surgery... It didn't matter what it was, he had it." Michael's nose began to collapse in after so many surgeries. Dr. Arnold Klein told Larry King in 2009, "I restored his nose with fillers. I tried hyaluronic acids, which were really effective. Because you don't want to put too much in, it's a difficult operation. And you must follow the instructions to the letter so that the material flows smoothly."

Admitting to having work done is one of the last big Hollywood taboos. Whether it is simply a little Botox or a more serious cosmetic operation like breast implants or a facelift, celebrities who have gone under the knife have remained in utter denial for a long time. However, times are changing, and a few courageous celebs are speaking up about their positive and negative experiences with plastic surgery and cosmetic injectables.

Here is what some celebrities had to say about cosmetic procedures:

In a cover story interview with InStyle in 2013, the singer Britney Spears discussed a little about aesthetic change.

"A doctor I visit (Beverly Hills plastic surgeon, Dr. Raj Kanodia), occasionally does fun stuff to me—I've had lip injections previously," she explained.

The Big Bang Theory star Kaley Cuoco revealed to Women's Health that she underwent a nose operation, breast augmentation ("the finest thing I ever did," she added), and fillers. "I'm sorry, but as much as you want to appreciate your inner self, you still want to look nice," she explained. "I don't believe you should do it for a guy or anybody else, but if it gives you confidence, that's fantastic."

"All of the fillers have been removed from my body. I'm the most natural person you'll ever meet," Courteney Cox told New Beauty in June 2017. "I feel better because I look like myself."

Kylie Jenner: Jenner disclosed that she underwent lip injections on her app. "Right now, all I have are lip fillers... But I'm also someone who believes in the phrase 'never say never.'

I'm not opposed to altering anything on my body if I come to a point where I'm truly uncomfortable with it," she wrote.

Cindy Crawford: "I'm not going to lie to myself: creams work on the texture of your skin beyond a certain age, but the only way to restore elasticity is with vitamin injections, Botox, and collagen," the model explained. "I live a very basic, healthy life that has worked wonders for me. I drink a lot of water, keep track of what I eat, and work out... My cosmetic surgeon, on the other hand, is responsible for the quality of my skin."

Cardi B: She discussed her breast augmentation and illicit butt injections (something you should never undertake; ramifications from illegal and so-called back-alley treatments can be catastrophic—even fatal). She was outspoken in 2019 about having liposuction and coming back to performing.

Ariel Winter: Winter revealed in 2015 that she had her breasts removed after years of physical and mental pain. "I purchased it for myself. I can't even put into words how fantastic it feels to feel completely at ease," she remarked.

Cosmetic surgery is in high demand, but what is the emotional impact of altering your appearance?

Social worker Roberta Honigman and psychiatrists Katharine Phillips, MD, and David Castle, MD, researched 37 studies on patients' psychological and psychosocial functioning before and after cosmetic surgery.

They found positive outcomes in patients, including improvements in body image and possibly a quality-of-life boost. However, the same study, which appeared in the April 2004 edition of Plastic and Reconstructive Surgery (Vol. 113, No. 4, pages 1,229-1,237), discovered significant predictors of poor results, particularly in individuals with high expectations or a history of melancholy and anxiety. Patients who are unhappy with their surgery may want repeat treatments, or they may face melancholy, adjustment issues, social isolation, familial troubles, self-destructive behaviours, and animosity against the surgeon and his/her team, according to the study. Men and women alike are growing more conscious about their physical appearance and pursuing cosmetic augmentation.

The majority of research shows that consumers are typically satisfied with the results of cosmetic treatments, although there has been little thorough testing.

More substantial (type change) treatments (e.g., rhinoplasty) seem to need more psychological adjustment on the part of the patients than 'restorative' surgeries (e.g., facelift). Patients who have unreasonable expectations about the outcome of cosmetic operations are more likely to be unhappy with the results.

Despite strong procedural outcomes, some people are never happy with aesthetic procedures. Some of them suffer from 'body dysmorphic disorder,' a psychological condition.

For a long time, my acquaintance would tell me that he was unhappy with his appearance and that he needed surgery to get his desired appearance. People still resort to cosmetic surgeons for penis lengthening, breast operations, or facelifts, and all of these procedures are typically an emotional decision resulting from a problem or perhaps a vocation in which they want to appear beautiful, especially if they are in the show business.

Finally, it is a choice one has to make. If you want to improve your appearance and a cosmetic surgeon is able to offer you that, you have to be prepared for the small chance that things may not go as planned. The end result may not live up to your expectations.

Plastic surgeons in the United States are well compensated and perform excellent work. They have greater experience as well; however, in India at this moment, plastic surgeons double up as cosmetic surgeons in their spare time and in their private clinics, while simultaneously doing plastic surgery and trauma surgery during the day. If you have to do a job that requires cosmetic surgery, then I recommend that you consult a surgeon who is well-versed in one form of surgery and likely specialises in it. If he is a cosmetic surgeon, he will be able to give you a top-class cosmetic procedure. However, do not expect all plastic surgeons to be able to perform top-notch cosmetic surgery procedures. A lot of people, both young and old, would like to get Botox.

This is usually done by surgeons, but it can also be done by cosmetologists, who are basically doctors who are not surgeons, but they have a good understanding of the anatomy of the face and would be able to do a good job. Look for individuals with a similar face form, who are close in age to you, and who share some of your worries. Surgery is a major thing, and the road to your new appearance can be a winding one. You must be completely at ease with your cosmetic surgeon and their support staff. Choose a cosmetic surgeon with whom you feel comfortable and to whom you can entrust your safety and results completely. Yes, it is quite natural to have some 'post-surgery' blues, sad sentiments, or emotions. The first few days after the surgery could be overwhelming as there is swelling around the operated part and it looks worse than it did before. The majority of emotional reactions to cosmetic surgery disappear rapidly as you begin to feel better during your recuperation. However, if mental distress persists for more than a few days or weeks, or if it is severe, consider counselling.

If you have complicated or unreasonable expectations about what surgery may do—such as believing it can save a broken relationship or turn your life around—you are choosing cosmetic surgery for the wrong reasons. During a consultation, it is critical to discuss your reasons and objectives for cosmetic surgery—as well as your expectations—with your surgeon, and to seek counselling if necessary.

There is progress in every area of the medical sciences and plastic surgery is no exception. After the full-face transplant, we are also looking at limb transplants from cadavers. Artificial skins grown in the labs are used to treat burn patients, while skin banks are developed around the world akin to the blood banks.

The more advanced cosmetic clinics around the world are providing a unique experience where the consulting rooms have multiple cameras to provide a 3D reconstruction of your image, like the one you would get after the proposed surgery!

All surgeries have their complication rates and so do plastic and cosmetic surgeries. A few may go really wrong and the patient may end up looking worse than before. A patient who underwent a breast lift complained that she was unable to sleep at night because her nipples were at different levels! Similarly, a patient who underwent penile implantation had to be admitted to the Emergency Department when he tried to test the results of the procedure before the healing process was complete! The penile implants were seen jetting out from the organ concerned and it was not a pretty sight! You should remember that all plastic surgeons really put their hearts into the procedures they do for their patients, but if you have any reservations about the complications, DO NOT GET IT DONE! Period!

The human body is a fragile combination of bones, muscles, and skin, and we never know when something unexpected may happen. If you or a loved one has suffered a catastrophic injury, it is critical to seek the help of a board-certified plastic surgeon who specialises in reconstructive surgery.

| Values | Credits | Surgeon A | Surgeon B | Surgeon C | Surgeon D | Surgeon E |
|---|---|---|---|---|---|---|
| Education | 1-4 | | | | | |
| Experience | 1-3 | | | | | |
| Availability | 1-3 | | | | | |
| Behavior | 1-3 | | | | | |
| Personality | 1-2 | | | | | |
| Word of mouth | 1-4 | | | | | |
| Internet likes | 1-2 | | | | | |
| Ikigai | 1-3 | | | | | |
| Written Testimonials | 1-2 | | | | | |
| Video Testimonials | 1-4 | | | | | |
| Total | | | | | | |

# 14
# WE KEEP IT THROBBING!
## Cardiovascular Surgery

*"Guard your heart above all else, for it determines the course of your life."* –
The Bible

For years, the field of cardiovascular surgery has been considered an exotic specialty, and those practicing in the field have been considered akin to Gods. It has been considered the ultimate pinnacle in the field of surgery.

The very term inspires awe and respect in our minds. Well, it is natural, considering how important a role we assign to the functioning of the heart. The biblical statement probably means something in a figurative way, but we would do well to take it in a literal sense as well. People in the older age groups might be familiar with the name of Dr. Christiaan Bernard, the heart surgeon from South Africa, who became renowned for performing the world's first heart transplant surgery. He performed the heart transplant operation on Louis Washkansky on December 3, 1967, at the Groote Schuur Hospital in Cape Town, South Africa. Closer home in India, Dr. KN Dastur performed the first open-heart surgery in the year 1961 at the Nair Hospital in Mumbai. A beating heart denotes life and hope.

It is a tangible sign that says we are still here and our time is not done yet. Dr. Mehmet Oz, a noted cardiothoracic surgeon and an American television personality, says, "…you have to be pretty arrogant to saw through a person's chest take out their heart and believe you can fix it."

Cardiovascular surgery, or the more inclusive term cardiothoracic and vascular surgery, deals with the surgical management of diseases that affect our cardiovascular system. This involves conditions affecting the heart, blood vessels, and lungs. A person suffering from any condition affecting these organs and requiring surgical treatment would have to visit a cardiovascular surgeon.

### Identify your surgeons

You would have noticed that there are three different terms in use here—Cardiac Surgeons, Thoracic Surgeons, and Vascular Surgeons. Although the field of surgery is interconnected among these three roles, and many of the surgeons might be performing overlapping roles, they do have a specific area in the cardiovascular system where they reign as the experts.

How can you choose or identify who is the best surgeon to treat your condition? To do that, you need to have a fair idea of what specific conditions each of these surgeons operate on or treat. And one should also be aware of the training that they undergo to become specialists in their chosen area. Unfortunately, in our country, we either have very well-known and prominent cardiovascular surgical specialists who are like stars and are greatly in demand due to their popularity and skills, or there are others who are considered to be mere assistants. This is somewhat akin to wealth distribution in our country. There is an 'all or none' status accorded to cardiovascular surgeons. Cardiac Surgeons primarily operate on the heart. They perform procedures such as open-heart surgery for heart transplantation, heart valve replacement surgeries, and cardiac bypass surgeries. They may also perform surgeries on structures or tissues that are immediately adjacent to the heart as well.

Thoracic surgeons, for the main part, operate on the lungs, which may be affected by cancers or other infectious conditions like Tuberculosis of the lung. These surgeons would have also been trained in performing cardiac surgeries as part of their specialty training, but they are more comfortable working with structures other than the heart. Sometimes thoracic surgeons might be general surgeons who have made thoracic surgery an area of their expertise. Cancer surgeons or Onco-surgeons, too, operate in the thoracic region in some circumstances. They perform surgeries in cases of tumours, such as chondromas or sarcomas.

Onco-surgeons might also perform lung resection in case of cancer in the lungs.

Vascular surgeons are trained to surgically manage diseases that involve the vast network of blood vessels in our bodies.

Let us take a detailed look at each of these surgical specialists and the work that they are trained to do. To start with, all surgeons will need to take the MS General Surgery training before being considered for the super-specialisation. Later they undergo further training in cardiovascular surgery and thus obtain the MCh. Degree in Cardio-Thoracic and Vascular surgery. A few institutes now offer only vascular surgery specialisations without the cardio-thoracic tag.

### Cardiac Surgeons

Cardiac surgeons are trained specifically to surgically treat disease conditions of the heart. Some of the procedures that they perform are explained here:

**Coronary Artery Bypass Grafting (CABG):** The term commonly used to refer to this procedure is 'Bypass surgery.' This procedure is used to treat coronary heart disease. The coronary arteries supply blood to the heart muscles. They may get occluded with a clot, or they may get narrowed in certain conditions. When the vessels are narrowed and there is decreased blood supply to the heart muscles, the patient can experience chest pain, called Angina. When there is a sudden loss of blood supply to a part of the heart muscle due to a clot blocking the blood vessel, the patient suffers a heart attack. In CABG, a section of a blood vessel from another part of the body, such as the chest or leg, is taken and attached to the affected coronary artery such that blood flow is diverted around the diseased or stenosed portion. The new section of blood vessel used is known as the 'graft.' This procedure can now be performed by opening the chest wall using a tiny incision. This is termed 'minimally invasive cardiac surgery' (MICS) or Robot-assisted cardiac surgery. The MICS and the Robotic procedures have the significant advantage of a faster recovery, but overall results may not differ between open-heart surgery and the MICS or Robotic surgeries.

**Valve Repair/Replacement Surgery:** The human heart has four valves that help in regulating the flow of blood between the chambers of the heart or through the major blood vessels leading from the heart. Sometimes these valves can get diseased and their function can be compromised. They may either become too wide in certain conditions or become very narrow in others. In such cases, cardiac surgeons either repair the damaged valve or replace the diseased valve if it is damaged extensively. These too can be done via the 'Open' method, MICS, or a Robot-assisted procedure. Robot-assisted surgeries are fast becoming very popular due to the significant precision that the robotic visualisation provides and flexibility of instrumentation that it offers, which finally result in better postoperative recovery and better overall results.

**Congenital Heart Disease Correction:** There are a number of congenital heart disorders that babies can be born with. You might have heard the term 'hole in the heart,' which is commonly used to refer to these conditions. Congenital heart disease affects the functioning of the heart and can have a negative effect on the child's growth and development. Sometimes these defects are mild, but often they are severe and need early surgical correction to restore the proper functioning of the heart.

Pediatric cardiac surgeons are specially trained to perform these delicate heart surgeries.

**Heart Transplantation:** In a heart transplantation procedure, the surgeon replaces the diseased or nonfunctional heart with a donor heart. The diseased heart is removed and the donor heart is sutured in place. The respective blood vessels are also sutured to the donor heart. The donor heart is usually received from a brain-dead patient.Heart transplantation surgeries are being performed for more than five decades now, and the recipient patients enjoy a good quality of life for many years after the surgery. The problem in these cases is the availability of donor organs. Recently, a genetically modified heart from a Pig was transplanted in a human, and that has shown promising results.

### Thoracic Surgeons

Thoracic surgeons are those who operate on the organs present in the chest cavity apart from the heart. These include the lungs, oesophagus (food pipe), trachea (windpipe), and other tissues and supporting structures present in the chest cavity. These surgeons could be cardio-thoracic super-specialists or simply general surgeons with specialist training. These surgeons are more interested in performing thoracic surgery alone and do not prefer to do cardiac surgeries. Some of the conditions that these surgeons treat are listed below:

**Lung cancer:** Lung resection may be indicated when patients suffer from cancer in the lung. A part of a lung or the whole lung may have to be removed.

Tuberculosis of the lung: The diseased section of the lung has to be resected in these patients. Surgery in the mediastinum and surgery on the thymus gland also fall under their domain.

**Vascular Surgeons**

Vascular surgeons treat diseases affecting the blood vessels—arteries and veins, and the lymphatic vessels in the rest of the body, except for those in the brain and the heart. These are taken care of by the neurosurgeons and the cardiac surgeons, respectively. Let us see some of the conditions that these surgeons treat.

**Abdominal Aortic Aneurysm:** The main aorta becomes thin-walled and bulges, and it might rupture at any time.

**Chronic arterial insufficiency:** There is decreased blood supply to an organ because of the narrowing of the blood vessel.

Lymphedema.

Varicose veins: This condition leads to swollen lower limbs.

Vascular infections.

Vascular trauma.

Blood clots in either the veins or arteries: This can cause the sudden death of an organ due to a lack of blood supply.

Vascular surgeons are trained to operate on the blood vessels in our body. They specialise in Vascular Surgery after completing postgraduate training in General Surgery. They are highly skilled in performing delicate procedures on even very small blood vessels. It is a highly demanding and tiring field.

They treat patients who have their arteries blocked due to a clot or an atheroma. An atheroma is a build-up of fatty deposits and other material in the inner layer of the blood vessels. These can block the blood flow and cause narrowing of the vessel, or they can break off and move away from the site of origin to cause a block elsewhere. Sometimes a person may faint suddenly and the cause may be a block or a stricture in one of the blood vessels in the neck. Blood vessels that run in the neck region are important because they supply blood to the brain. Vascular surgeons operate to restore normal blood flow in the affected blood vessel.

Vascular surgeons also treat Aneurysms of the aorta or other big arteries. An aneurysm occurs when there is a weakening of a section of a wall of the artery causing that portion to bulge or balloon out. Aneurysms occur most commonly in the aorta. They may occur in the brain as well, but these are treated by neurosurgeons. Aneurysms need to be treated as an emergency because they may burst at any time and are potentially life-threatening.

In certain disease conditions, the blood flow to the limbs, especially the legs, may be compromised. This may be due to an acute cause like atherosclerosis or a blood clot. Patients with longstanding uncontrolled Diabetes can also present with vascular compromise in the lower limbs. Or it may involve a chronic condition such as varicose veins, where the return of the blood from the legs to the heart is impaired due to inefficient valves in the veins. Blood clots in the blood vessels supplying the intestines or lungs are potentially life-threatening. If the clot is not removed and the blood supply restored immediately, these organs can suffer irreversible damage, sometimes even leading to the death of the individual.

Vascular surgeons can treat all these conditions, and they help preserve the limb or leg, which might, if left untreated, even end up getting amputated to save the life of the patient.

Another area where vascular surgeons are often called upon is trauma surgery. Road traffic accidents and other incidents of trauma can cause arteries and veins to be cut or damaged. Vascular surgeons play a huge role in these situations where they repair and anastomose the torn blood vessels to restore blood flow. Another area where vascular surgeons are called upon is when the patient develops blood clots either without any cause or after an unrelated surgery. These clots usually develop in the legs and can travel up into the brain or the lungs and are potentially life-threatening.

Many newer vascular surgeons are doing Endo-vascular work akin to what cardiologists call percutaneous transluminal coronary angioplasty (PTCA) and stenting. The difference is that the cardiologist carries out the procedure in the vessels of the heart while the vascular surgeons do it in the vessels in other parts of the body.

Essentially, it involves going into the affected vessels through a puncture in the skin using a very fine tube, injecting a dye, identifying the block in the artery of interest, and finally placing a stent to bridge the narrowing; this serves to restore normal blood supply to the affected organs. Being a minimal access surgery, this procedure has benefits such as less bleeding and lesser chances of infection with better healing. For stenting procedures on blocked arteries, they use a C-Arm and inject dye to locate the block. The C-Arm is a movable imaging unit used in cardiac or orthopaedic surgeries. It allows the surgeon to visualise the images on a screen. The procedure is quick and results in the patient being up and about in a couple of days. That is definitely a good development because back when stents were not available and the image-guided stenting procedure was yet to be developed, treating these patients would involve making a large incision and the patient would need to be hospitalised for many days.

As you can see, vascular surgeons attend to emergencies most of the time. Their skills are invaluable in saving lives. They need to be on call 24/7 and hardly get any rest. They work untiringly, and I often feel sorry for them because they work so hard. Only in a few situations, such as varicose vein surgery, do vascular surgeons perform elective procedures. All the rest are emergency procedures calling for a high degree of skill and dedication.

While talking about cardiovascular surgeries, the most common term you would have heard would be open-heart surgery. However, the latest developments in this field involve minimally invasive procedures. Let us learn a little more about these.

## Open-heart Surgery Versus Minimally Invasive Procedures

In a previous section, we looked at the various operations that cardiac surgeons perform on the heart. The heart is present in the thoracic cavity behind the ribs, on the left side. Traditionally, heart surgeries have been done by cutting through the sternum or the breast bone.

This allows the surgeon to access the heart and its blood vessels. This procedure was termed 'open-heart surgery,' where 'open' referred to the chest wall. This was a major surgical procedure and the pain associated with it was severe.

The sternum is considered one of the most painful parts of the body and the healing of the sternum is very slow. However, in the open-heart procedure, the surgeon has a good view of the field and can be sure of operating accurately. Especially in cardiac bypass surgery, the advantages of this procedure are the slightly lower cost and maybe better longevity of the graft.

The disadvantages would be the larger incision involving a longer healing time and a longer hospital stay.

The new revolution in the field of surgery is the development of minimal access surgery in all specialties. In cardiac surgery, too, Minimally Invasive Cardiac Surgeries (MICS) are now being performed by some cardiac surgeons.

In MICS, the cardiac surgeons have gone beyond the sternal splitting procedure, where the sternum has to be resected to reach the heart. They now access the heart through a small space between the ribs, and they are able to do the same procedures that were traditionally performed by the open-heart method. MICS has changed the way patients perceive heart surgeries completely.

MICS is considered a very good alternative to open-heart surgery. It appears to have many advantages over open-heart surgeries.

In general, it has been reported that minimally invasive procedures make a huge difference in terms of patient recovery. Patients undergoing MICS recover from the procedure faster than those who undergo the traditional open-heart procedure. The pain is less and also recovery is quicker. The patient has a lesser hospital and ICU stay as well.

However, the cost of MICS is definitely higher, but patients might consider it a small price to pay for the benefits they get in experiencing less pain and a faster recovery. However, one has to think of the actual procedure. Cardiovascular surgery is not a cosmetic procedure; rather, it is a life-saving surgery.

For instance, if you have been diagnosed with a blocked coronary artery and been advised to undergo a cardiac bypass graft surgery, which would you choose? A costlier procedure that has the benefits of less pain and shorter hospitalisation, but requires a greater effort and skill of the surgeon and is performed with lesser access? Or the tried and tested open-heart surgery where the pain is greater and the hospital stay is longer, but has a lot of older surgeons who are trained to do it well.

Ultimately, any life-saving procedure that you choose should give you better and longer-lasting results than the other options. In this situation, it would mean the longevity of the graft. A 30-year follow-up study of patients who underwent CABG reports the median life expectancy to be 17.6 years. Does MICS give a better result or improved longevity?

The fact is, there are not many studies or double-blind trials reported comparing the results of these two surgical techniques. MICS might seem to have numerous benefits like a shorter hospital stay, faster recovery, lesser blood loss, and smaller incisions, but there is a long way to go before it is accepted as the front runner or gold standard when it comes to cardiac surgeries, especially for bypass surgeries.

The reason I say this is not because the efficacy and superiority of MICS have been unproved yet; rather, not enough surgeons have adopted this procedure.

There is a lack of sufficient data to come to a conclusion, although emerging evidence points toward MICS having the same outcomes at early and medium terms.

Without sufficient data, it is difficult to say which procedure is better. The same applies to surgery on the valves of the heart as well. I know some of my medical colleagues who underwent open-heart valvular surgery on the advice of their surgeons. However, the same surgeons opted to undergo a MICS procedure for themselves. This ambiguity in deciding the treatment of choice is simply due to a lack of data availability.

The situation is similar to what happened in the case of cardiac stents. Coronary stents are basically elongated tube-like devices, which are placed in arteries that have developed a blockage or are narrowed with strictures. The stent opens up the artery and restores normal blood flow.

At one time, absorbable stents were in use, and they were highly in vogue. However, with time they were withdrawn from use because they did not prove their worth. They did not efficiently perform the job they were meant to.

Another development in the field of surgery is robotic surgery or robotic-assisted surgery. Some surgeons have started performing robotic-assisted procedures in cardiac surgeries as well. The same procedures that were done through MICS are now being done robotically.

It certainly has advantages like providing the surgeon with a better vision and permitting extremely dexterous movements of the hands.

It does seem poised to take off in a big way, but sooner or later, with enough data, we will come to know if there is a price to pay for it.

Vascular surgeons, too, are increasingly adopting the use of minimally invasive procedures in their field. Therefore, I would say minimally invasive procedures are good and welcome, but the surgeon and the patient should decide which is a better option. This depends on the severity and extent of the disease, position of the block, co-morbidities present in the patient, expertise of the surgeon, etc.

There are cardiac surgeons, thoracic surgeons, and vascular surgeons. They each have their own field of expertise. There might be some common procedures that they all can perform with competence, some overlap in their roles. However, you should be aware of what your disease or problem is and then consult the appropriate surgeon for treatment. I say this because the surgeon who specialises in a particular field will have the necessary experience after having performed numerous similar surgeries over the years.

I also say, tongue-in-cheek, that most of these surgeons would also like to do the other guy's job, but it might not be their best effort due to lack of experience or a half-hearted approach!

| Values | Credits | Surgeon A | Surgeon B | Surgeon C | Surgeon D | Surgeon E |
|---|---|---|---|---|---|---|
| Education | 1-4 | | | | | |
| Experience | 1-3 | | | | | |
| Availability | 1-3 | | | | | |
| Behavior | 1-3 | | | | | |
| Personality | 1-2 | | | | | |
| Word of mouth | 1-4 | | | | | |
| Internet likes | 1-2 | | | | | |
| Ikigai | 1-3 | | | | | |
| Written Testimonials | 1-2 | | | | | |
| Video Testimonials | 1-4 | | | | | |
| Total | | | | | | |

# 15
# THE LIGHT IN YOUR LIFE AND THE MUSIC IN YOUR EARS!
### Ophthalmology & Otorhinolaryngology

### Who are the Ophthalmologists?

Ophthalmologists are doctors who have specialised in the diagnosis and treatment of conditions and diseases that affect our eyes. Everybody, at some time or the other, would have made a visit to an eye doctor. They play a very crucial role in keeping our vision sharp. You would have come across many terms in relation to the eye specialist: Ophthalmologist, Optometrist, and Optician. Do they mean the same? No! Each of these is a different professional, although all three are involved in providing eye care to patients. The difference between them lies in the level of training and expertise and also in the conditions that they specifically cater to. Optometrists are trained in diagnosing and managing refractive errors. They are not medical doctors, but they have a degree in optometry and can accurately check your eyes and provide corrective spectacles or glasses as required.

They also would be familiar with eye diseases and can direct you to an ophthalmologist for care. Optometrists can write out eyeglass prescriptions.

Oculists are mainly involved in verifying and fitting patients with corrective eyeglasses and contact lenses. They do not by themselves check a patient's vision or prescribe eyeglasses, but they use the prescriptions provided by the ophthalmologists and optometrists to provide patients with the correct lenses and glasses. They do not diagnose or treat any eye diseases.

Ophthalmologists are doctors who have specialized in the medical and surgical treatment of eye conditions. They would have acquired their postgraduate training in MS Ophthalmology after completing their MBBS course. They can also complete the Diplomate in National Board (DNB) exam in ophthalmology to get their specialisation. They take care of all the medical and surgical issues with the eyes. They can diagnose and treat all eye diseases, perform different types of eye surgeries, and prescribe corrective glasses and lenses for vision problems (refractive errors) as well.

In general, ophthalmologists are considered the most petite and delicate surgeons in the hospital. After all, they deal with one of the most delicate structures in the body—the eye! And ophthalmology is a rapidly developing branch with new advances in treatments made almost every day.

So, what are the conditions that ophthalmologists treat? Well, they may be classified as emergency conditions, routine outpatient cases, and of course eye surgeries. The most frequently seen emergency conditions involving the eye would be a foreign body on the cornea or trauma to the eye. As a person's vision is at stake here, prompt treatment is required in these cases. Ophthalmologists treat a whole lot of cases in their OPDs, from infections to refractive errors. Prescribing corrective glasses and lenses is a major part of what they do. The ophthalmologist tests your vision and gives you the proper eyeglasses to see clearly. From the young to the old, these days everyone definitely makes a visit to their ophthalmologist for checking their vision and getting it rectified.

Older people need reading glasses due to a condition called Presbyopia. Without near vision glasses, older folks cannot read or do work that requires accurate near vision.

Now, patients may have defective vision due to causes other than refractive errors. A lot of systemic health conditions like diabetes and hypertension cause problems in the eye. These conditions when untreated can cause irreversible loss of vision. The eye doctor can look into your eyes and tell you if your blood sugar or your blood pressure is under control. They dilate the eye and use a scope called an ophthalmoscope to look at the retina. So, what can you expect when you visit an ophthalmologist? Usually, these guys dilate the pupil of the eye. This can take 30 minutes to 2 hours. When your pupils are dilated, your vision would be blurry, and it will be dangerous for you to drive back from the doctor's office. It is often advised to take someone with you to drive you back.

The eye is basically a window into the whole body. Various changes in the retina allow the eye surgeon to diagnose conditions like diabetic retinopathy, hypertensive retinopathy, and even problems in the brain. If there is a tumour in the brain causing raised pressure inside the brain, this can be diagnosed by viewing the optic nerve in the retina.

Some patients have defective vision because of retinal detachment. The retina is avulsed completely or the patient may have holes in the retina. This can cause defective vision. Or the pressure in the eye per se can be raised due to blockage of ducts or other reasons. This condition is called glaucoma. If untreated, this can again cause blindness in the patient. One of the main reasons for decreased vision or loss of vision in older people is cataracts. Almost all old people will need to make a visit to their eye doctor to assess their cataracts and to decide when to have them operated on. This is one of the main surgeries that ophthalmologists perform. Along with the correction of refractive errors, cataract surgeries form their bread and butter. And cataracts can sometimes occur in young people as well, especially as a result of penetrating trauma to the eye.

Conditions like Glaucoma and Diabetic Retinopathy are called silent killers. In the initial phase of the disease, the condition may not incapacitate you so much, but as it progresses, it may cause permanent damage to the eye and result in complete blindness. Hence, if you have diabetes or a family history of glaucoma, or you are above 50 years of age, it is important to get your eyes checked annually so that these conditions can be diagnosed early and treated.

It is especially important after the pandemic, where everything else tends to be neglected, apart from the Corona virus-related maladies.

Ophthalmic surgeries are very intricate. There are different types of cataract surgeries, each one more evolved or advanced than the previous one. The most recent development in cataract surgeries is the Phaco procedure. The complete term is 'phacoemulsification' with intraocular lens (IOL) implantation. As the term suggests, the cataractous lens is removed and an artificial lens is implanted. The incision used in this procedure is extremely tiny and these incisions are self-sealing; there are no sutures used. The wound heals quickly and the patient has a faster recovery as well. These days technology has advanced to the extent that the patient's vision can be corrected by implanting a lens with the correct power at the time of cataract surgery. This means that a patient who used to wear glasses for vision before he/she developed a cataract can get normal vision following IOL implantation, provided their cornea and retina are normal.

Every eye surgeon on completing their Postgraduate degree will be proficient in performing these cataract surgeries and also other ophthalmic surgical procedures, such as foreign body removal, trabeculectomy (to treat glaucoma), or dacryocystorhinostomy (to treat blocked tear ducts). However, there are some areas in ophthalmology that require specialised training. Ophthalmologists undergo special training in various types of procedures depending on which segment of the eye interests them. Those who undergo training in posterior segment diseases are experts in treating conditions that affect the retina. They are trained in using Laser therapy. Laser treatments are used in the management of conditions like diabetic retinopathy, retinal tears, or retinal detachment.

Laser therapy is also used to treat glaucoma by a procedure called laser trabeculectomy.

Some ophthalmologists get trained in the treatment of congenital conditions of the eye, such as squint. Early surgical correction of the squint is vital for the child to have normal vision in the affected eye. Eye surgeons trained in squint corrective surgeries perform these procedures.

A procedure that is now becoming very popular among the younger crowd is the LASIK procedure. It stands for Laser-Assisted In-Situ Keratomileusis. This is a surgical procedure used to permanently correct refractive errors in younger patients. Those who have been wearing eyeglasses since childhood and want to be rid of their burden opt to undergo this procedure. The LASIK machine is a large one, and here a specialised laser beam is used to make calculated cuts in the cornea to thin it out and thereby correct the refractive error. Normal vision is restored and the patient does not need to wear glasses thereafter.

Now that you have an idea of the different conditions that can affect the eye, it is easy to decide whom to consult. In case of an emergency, such as a foreign body in the eye, trauma, or sudden loss of vision, one should go to the nearest ophthalmologist or multispeciality hospital where you are sure to have an eye surgeon on call.

For routine OPD consultations, choose an eye clinic or hospital that is clean and has a regular ophthalmologist seeing the patients. You need to be sure that you are not consulting an optometrist.

For cataract surgeries, most specialist eye hospitals have eye surgeons trained in phaco surgeries and you can find the ophthalmologist you want to consult based on reviews and by asking your friends and relatives who have undergone cataract surgeries. If a hospital has a phaco machine, then the surgeon would be trained and competent to perform the procedure.

It is best to consult eye surgeons trained in posterior segment procedures for the management of diseases like diabetic retinopathy and other retinal conditions.

These specialists are usually present in Multispeciality Hospitals or Speciality Eye Hospitals.

For all paediatric eye problems, like congenital anomalies or squint correction, it is best to consult eye surgeons specially trained in these procedures. With the increased use of gadgets, children as well as adults are increasingly developing eye issues, which makes it extremely important to visit your ophthalmologist regularly for an eye evaluation. You may find nothing, but believe me, it is worth a visit!

Lasik is a fully automated procedure and there is not much room for manmade errors. However, choose a hospital where they have been doing the procedure for a few years with good results. Also, ensure that you can afford the cost of the procedure. One of the main things to look out for, whatever the procedure you are going in for, is the cleanliness of the hospital.

## Otorhinolaryngology

The ENT specialists have a very fancy name: Otorhinolaryngologist. But they are commonly just known as ENT surgeons or sometimes just plain ENTs. In fact, these are the only guys who are called just by the organs they treat! Even the ophthalmologist gets referred to as the eye doctor and not the 'eye.'

There is a common perception that an ENT specialist treats allergies, ear infections, and tonsil problems. However, these are just a few basic conditions that these specialists treat. They are trained for so much more and they are indeed doing so much more in their field. How does one get qualified as an ENT specialist? An aspiring ENT surgeon takes up MS ENT or DNB ENT after completion of the MBBS course. A qualified ENT surgeon can perform surgeries and medically treat conditions pertaining to the ear, nose, and throat regions. All of us would have visited an ENT specialist at some point in our lives for the treatment of conditions ranging from sniffles, coughs, and colds to ear pain and throat pain. Indeed, these were the conditions that were commonly treated by these guys in earlier times.

Their OPDs were usually very busy as these are common ailments in people and there would be many patients.

Most of these conditions were caused by underlying infections and therefore could be treated in the OPD itself. The specialty has evolved and grown over the years. ENT specialists now manage a lot more than the traditional ear, nose, and throat cases. Nowadays, they also treat various conditions pertaining to the head and neck regions. This includes the diseases of the thyroid gland and cancers that occur in the neck region or cancers in the mouth and tongue.

If you were to look at a typical sample of patients attending an ENT OPD at the present time, you are likely to see patients with the following conditions:

- Ear problems such as pain, infections, loss of hearing, ringing in the ears, and loss of balance.
- Allergies, sinus infections, and growths in the nasal cavity.
- Tonsil problems, difficulty in swallowing, sore throat, or a change in voice.
- Breathing difficulties or excessive snoring or choking evidence in the night.
- Tumours in the head and neck region.

So, there is a wide gamut of conditions that they look into in this area.

The ENT specialists have been operating in the ear, nose, and throat areas for a while now, and it was just a matter of time before they took the next logical step of operating on the head and neck regions as well as they are quite familiar with these areas too.

The ENT specialists are specially trained to diagnose and treat paediatric ENT conditions. Very young children will not be able to tell what is ailing them or where they are experiencing pain or discomfort. They may have an infection or it might just be impacted wax. As soon as the wax is removed, pain is relieved and hearing is restored! The other conditions that they treat include middle ear infections and eardrum ruptures.

If we were to look at the emergencies seen in ENT practice, among children, the commonest would be a foreign body in the ear canal or nostril.

These children would be brought in by the parents in a panic, and the ENT surgeon can remove these foreign bodies using special forceps or other instruments. Other emergencies seen would be bleeding from the nose as a result of trauma or a nasal polyp, obstruction to the airway caused by anaphylaxis, or an inhaled foreign body.

There have been awesome advances in ENT techniques in recent times. One such area where there is path-breaking progress is in the management of congenital anomalies in children. Children with certain congenital diseases have complete hearing loss. One example of this is congenital external auditory canal atresia.

The new technique used to restore hearing in these children is called BAHA—Bone Anchored Hearing Aid. BAHA is extremely beneficial to those having ear canal atresia or chronic ear discharge due to infection. ENT surgeons undergo special training to become competent in this technique, but the smiles on the faces of children and their parents are worth any trouble.

It is indeed special to see the child's face when he can hear the mother's voice for the first time, and the mother's happiness knows no bounds either when the child hears her for the first time. These are special moments in their field.

The other specialised area in ENT practice is Cochlear implants. These are electronic devices that are used when the inner ear mechanism is not functioning either from birth or due to some other reason. Cochlear implants restore hearing in these patients. However, if the hearing loss is from birth, a cochlear implant gives the best results when the procedure is performed before the age of five to six years. This procedure is very expensive, and the surgeon who performs the implant procedure would be a well-trained expert as the accurate placement of the electrodes is very important.

When it comes to diseases affecting the nose, the common conditions are sinusitis, nasal polyps, and deviated nasal septum.

Surgical management of these conditions is a lot less traumatic these days because of the use of endoscopic techniques.

Endoscopic sinus surgery aids in relieving symptoms caused by sinusitis and nasal polyps, nasal obstruction, nasal tumours, etc. The procedure is a minimally invasive technique and is termed Functional Endoscopic Sinus Surgery (FESS). FESS is used these days to restore sinus ventilation and normal function. FESS aids in reducing the number and severity of sinus infections and improving airflow through the nose, symptoms associated with sinusitis, and the sense of smell.

Many of these ENT surgeons who have been trained in endoscopic procedures are so good that they assist neurosurgeons when they have to operate on the base of the skull to remove the cribriform plate.

The cribriform plate is a thin bone that separates the sinuses from the brain and the pituitary gland. There is indeed an increasing cross-over seen these days as surgeons of different specialities help each other achieve the best possible outcomes for the patients. Here, the ENT endoscopic surgeons help the neurosurgeons operate on the pituitary gland by providing access. Of course, they do not operate on the pituitary gland themselves.

Operations on the throat are mainly performed for tonsillitis and adenoiditis. Chronic inflammation of the adenoid glands is called adenoiditis, and this condition can cause sleep disturbances in children. Usually, these children are repeatedly seen in paediatric OPDs and then are referred to the ENT specialists for undergoing tonsillectomy or adenoidectomy, as the case may be.

So, who is a Head and Neck surgeon? An ENT specialist who is interested in head and neck surgery usually has to spend a lot of time working with an oncosurgeon who operates extensively in the head and neck region. Surgery in this area requires a lot of expertise and experience because the neck is a vital region. There are a lot of blood vessels traversing the neck region and operating in this area carries a huge risk. Only an experienced and well-trained surgeon would venture into this area.

Head and neck surgeons take care of conditions like muscle mass or tumour in the cheek or mouth and cancer in the vocal cords, thyroid, and parathyroid, among others. As far as routine ENT problems are concerned, you can consult an ENT surgeon who would be competent to deal with them.

They can deal with conditions such as eardrum perforations, routine sinus surgeries, and tonsillectomies. However, for specialized procedures like BAHA, Cochlear Implants, skull base surgeries, or Head and Neck surgeries, you should consult surgeons who have specialized in these respective fields.

They are basically ENT surgeons who have chosen a special area of interest—they find their ikigai—and they focus on this particular area and get trained in it. With years of experience, they become very good at what they do.

So, if you need surgical treatment in any of these areas, your best bet would be an organ-specific surgeon.

There are certain areas where ophthalmologists and ENT surgeons work together. There are several disorders that involve areas pertaining to both these specialities. Some of these conditions are orbital complications of sinusitis, exophthalmos, lacrimal gland and duct issues, tumours or trauma involving the eye and the face, optic nerve decompression, etc.

Of course, it is in the patient's interests for both the specialists to consult and share their knowledge, experience, and approaches, and this helps them achieve the best clinical end point.

# INCISIONS

| Values | Credits | Surgeon A | Surgeon B | Surgeon C | Surgeon D | Surgeon E |
|---|---|---|---|---|---|---|
| Education | 1-4 | | | | | |
| Experience | 1-3 | | | | | |
| Availability | 1-3 | | | | | |
| Behavior | 1-3 | | | | | |
| Personality | 1-2 | | | | | |
| Word of mouth | 1-4 | | | | | |
| Internet likes | 1-2 | | | | | |
| Ikigai | 1-3 | | | | | |
| Written Testimonials | 1-2 | | | | | |
| Video Testimonials | 1-4 | | | | | |
| Total | | | | | | |

# REFERENCES

1. https://openmd.com/define?q=laparoscopic

2. https://www.sciencedirect.com/science/article/pii/S2444866416300186

3. https://mccartyweightloss.com/are-bariatric-surgery-cosmetic-surgery-the-same

4. https://www.osfhealthcare.org/blog/what-are-the-three-different-types-of-weight-loss-surgery/

5. https://www.osfhealthcare.org/blog/what-are-the-three-different-types-of-weight-loss-surgery/

6. https://www.theossi.com/guidelines-obesity-surgery.html

7. https://www.expresshealthcare.in/news/icmr-releases-data-on-incidence-rate-of-prostate-cancer-in-india/414265

8. https://pubmed.ncbi.nlm.nih.gov/26791046/

9. https://timesofindia.indiatimes.com/sports/cricket/news/bcci-wants-hub-for-sports-medicine-research-at-proposed-centre-of-excellence/articleshow/68161803.cms)

10. Verhey JT, Haglin JM, Verhey EM, Hartigan DE. Virtual, augmented, and mixed reality applications in orthopedic surgery. Int J Med Robot. 2020;16(2):e2067. doi:10.1002/rcs.2067

11. https://www.cancer.gov/about-cancer/treatment/types/surgery/lasers

# ABOUT THE AUTHOR

Dr. Saurabh Misra has been a practicing Consultant Gastrointestinal, Robotic and Bariatric surgeon at Apollo Hospitals in Bangalore since January 2007. He has been a surgeon since 1994 and seems to have improved in flavour and texture since his passing out from RNT medical college at Udaipur in Rajasthan India in 1997. He has conducted more than 9000 independent surgeries during these 28 years as a surgeon. He has served as a national faculty for the OSSI (Obesity Society of India) at various national and international conferences, including AIIMS (All India Institute of Medical Sciences, New Delhi).

He represented South India on the executive council of the Hernia Society of India. He is presently serving as the faculty for HIS (Hernia Society of India), APHS (Asia Pacific Hernia Society), and the AWR (Abdominal Wall Repair) which is the international group dedicated to surgery of complex hernia repair and abdominal wall reconstruction and OSSI (Obesity society of India).

He is the Fellow of the International College of surgeons and the Indian Association of Gastrointestinal Endo surgeons. He has more than 25 research papers presented at the national, international Conferences and indexed journals, to his credit on Minimal Access Surgery.

www.ingramcontent.com/pod-product-compliance
Lightning Source LLC
Chambersburg PA
CBHW030009290326
41934CB00005B/269